The Creative Arts in Palliative Care

by the same editor

Social Work in the British Isles
Edited by Malcolm Payne and Steven M. Shardlow
ISBN 978 1 85302 833 5

of related interest

Dying, Bereavement and the Healing Arts
Edited by Gillie Bolton
ISBN 978 1 84310 516 9

The Expressive Arts Activity Book
A Resource for Professionals
Suzanne Darley and Wende Heath
Foreword by Gene D. Cohen MD PhD
Illustrated by Mark Darley
ISBN 978 1 84310 861 0

Palliative Care, Social Work and Service Users
Making Life Possible
Peter Beresford, Lesley Adshead and Suzy Croft
ISBN 978 1 84310 465 0

Supporting the Child and the Family in Paediatric Palliative Care
Erica Brown with Brian Warr
Foreword by Dr. Sheila Shribman, National Clinical Director for Children,
Maternity Services, Department of Health
ISBN 978 1 84310 181 9

Empowering Children through Art and Expression
Culturally Sensitive Ways of Healing Trauma and Grief
Bruce St Thomas and Paul Johnson
ISBN 978 1 84310 789 7

Music Therapy in Children's Hospices
Jessie's Fund in Action
Edited by Mercédès Pavlicevic
Foreword by Victoria Wood
ISBN 978 1 84310 254 0

Music Therapy in Palliative Care
New Voices
Edited by David Aldridge
ISBN 978 1 85302 739 0

The Creative Arts in Palliative Care

Edited by Nigel Hartley and Malcolm Payne

Jessica Kingsley Publishers
London and Philadelphia

First published in 2008
by Jessica Kingsley Publishers
116 Pentonville Road
London N1 9JB, UK
and
400 Market Street, Suite 400
Philadelphia, PA 19106, USA

www.jkp.com

Copyright © Jessica Kingsley Publishers 2008

Library of Congress Cataloging in Publication Data
A CIP catalog record for this book is available from the Library of Congress

British Library Cataloguing in Publication Data
A CIP catalogue record for this book is available from the British Library

ISBN 978 1 84310 591 6

Printed and bound in Great Britain by
Athenaeum Press, Gateshead, Tyne and Wear

Contents

List of boxes and figures

Acknowledgements

All the contributors would like to thank the patients, families, visitors and staff who contributed to their work and studies; working with them has been a privilege. Thanks and acknowledgements are also given to colleagues and clinical supervisors for their support, insight and encouragement and to Arts Council England and the Alfred and Peggy Harvey Charitable Trust, the D'oyly Carte Charitable Trust, the David Butler Trust, the St. James's Place Foundation, the Corinne Burton Trust, the Daisy Foundation, Barclay's Community Fund and Croydon Council for their financial support towards developing some of the ideas and practical work covered in this book. Personal thanks go to Rachel Verney, Gary Ansdell and the late Michele Angelo Petrone for their input on study days at St Christopher's Hospice and to Thomas Travitzky. Finally, the editors are grateful for the support of St Christopher's Hospice and its chief executive, Barbara Monroe.

Part I

Developing Creative Arts in Palliative Care

1 Introduction – The Creative Arts in Palliative Care

Nigel Hartley and Malcolm Payne

In this book we share some experiences of, and demonstrate the value of, incorporating the creative arts into palliative care services. We also ask questions about the place of both artists and the arts in society and examine some of the issues that arise when attempting to integrate them into such healthcare settings.

Palliative care as a setting for creative arts

In the UK, palliative care is delivered from hospices, mostly fairly small independent charities with a loyalty to local communities and the need to engage support from them. Their independence, from official restrictions, as voluntary or third sector organisations, can provide a flexible and supportive environment for introducing innovations such as creative arts into palliative care. On the other hand, their size means that resources may be constrained to a focus on the main requirements of palliative care service provision, and creative arts may seem low priority. Local funders and supporters, thinking mainly about medical and nursing care of dying people, may not be able to imagine what the arts might offer.

Increasingly, palliative care teams operate as part of general hospitals, and palliative care will in the future be delivered in care homes. While creative arts and arts therapies have a foothold in healthcare, the palliative care role is often medical and nursing consultancy to specialist teams, so a creative arts contribution may be less practicable than in a specialised institution, such as a hospice.

Most people would like to die in their own homes, but a high proportion in some parts of the country are admitted to accident and emergency units in large hospitals and die there. Art and craft may be part of someone's home life, but illness may cut people off from the support and resources to pursue the arts.

The difficulties for the arts in every palliative care setting suggests that considerable commitment will be needed to find a role, initiate a service and develop its potential. We aim in this chapter to focus on the reasons for expending the energy and effort to invoke the arts in palliative care settings.

Commentary on the objectives of creative arts services in palliative care suggests that there are four main reasons for including them in the overall service:

- Art and creative work are a vital human activity (Shaw 1999). This objective sees art and creative activity as integral to a good quality of life and therefore appropriate as an element in a service that seeks to provide such a good quality of life for people approaching death. McLoughlin (1997, p.9) also expresses this objective in saying that the main purpose of a creative writing group in a day centre is 'to promote enjoyment of literature' and in another account, 'to help patients discover what themes and images are important to them' (McLoughlin 1995). A similar objective is found in the work of Rosetta Life (2007), which uses digital resources as a basis for communication and image-building.

- Art and creative work enhance emotional stability, personal enrichment and self-fulfilment (Kennett 2001).

- Art and creative work can offer a diversion from depression or difficulty. This objective is sometimes rejected as a purpose for creative work, for example by Gibson (1995), on the grounds that day care provision should have an active treatment philosophy.

- The arts as a therapy – both social and psychological (Aldridge 1998). This approach sees art as a phenomenological creative process enabling therapeutic interactions to take place, focusing on the development of hope and meaning in traumatic situations.

To sum these points up, if palliative care is about living life to the full, then that life will include the arts. We recognise this by enabling people to use television and radio, where artists and journalists constantly create extremely highquality experiences for people to watch, listen to and be stimulated by. Television and radio are so ubiquitous, we forget the quality of the work they display every moment of the day – even if we might criticise some of it as not to our taste. We recognise the importance of the arts by offering people pictures or flower arrangements or attractive views for their rooms or bedsides, and by providing an attractive natural environment in hospice or hospital gardens. All of these efforts are about offering patients aesthetic experiences, and we accept that a pleasing environment offers stability, enrichment and fulfilment. How much more fulfilling it can be to enable people to contribute to that environment. The chapters in Part II of this book demonstrate that the feedback about the provision of creative arts therapies in palliative care from patients and their families is almost universally one of pleasure. For staff trying to do a complex and difficult task, for families experiencing an important part of their life together, the arts are an instrument of motivation and experience. Moreover, in cases that are appropriate, they can be an important psychological therapy.

Although many artists employed to work in hospices will be based within day care facilities, this is not a book about day care only. The growing need to deliver effective palliative care in a wide range of community settings such as care homes and GP surgeries, and the current emphasis on public education, offer new possibilities for practising the arts, which we expand upon in Chapter 4, on exhibiting, promoting and funding the arts in healthcare, and in Chapters 11–13 on various aspects of the community arts in palliative care. Unlike much healthcare, which has taken place in large hospitals with an emphasis on bio-medical science in medical treatments and nursing care, palliative care incorporates strong elements of spiritual care and social work and welfare practice along with biomedical science; this, too offers an important context for arts work.

Palliative care brings to the arts the opportunity to interact with physical and mental deterioration, death, pain and loss. Arts practitioners in palliative care are present at a crucial transition in the lives of most families, shaped by powerful emotions and new personal, relationship and social experiences for patients and their families. All this can bring inspiration and stimulation to artists, and generate important opportunities for new artistic expression. It also brings the opportunity to demonstrate how the arts can help people deal with distress and difficulty; we can extend this learning from palliative care to other situations where people experience social and biomedical distress. People who experience the arts in this setting at this moment in their life experience may come to understand how they may participate in the arts more actively to better strengthen their resilience in dealing with future life experiences. They may increase the perception of the value of the arts in society. Through appreciating the contribution of the arts in palliative care, awareness might grow about what the arts can contribute to society in other areas, not just in health and social care; people might be drawn to support the arts in other aspects of their lives.

What can the arts and skilled, creative artists bring to a palliative care setting? Death, dying and bereavement are an important part of life, and while we all know that we will face them, we often do not think through our responses to these powerful elements of life in advance. The arts are a mechanism for facilitating a response to current experience and giving it meaning. Stanworth (2003), for example, in examining metaphor and image as a way of expressing the experience of dying among hospice patients, drew much of her analysis from patients' artwork. Using the creative arts with people facing death, dying and all that this brings is not just about offering them a 'nice time' or about 'taking their minds off their illness'. The arts bring with them possibilities; possibilities for motivation and growth, for coping and change, for self-actualisation and self-realisation. They also offer possibilities to make sense of situations, to create something of value and to leave something behind which says 'this was me, this is what my life has meant'. Those possibilities are not only for patients, but also for their families and carers. The second part of this book tells us stories of people whose lives have been changed through using the creative arts.

The arts move us. We all respond to them in one way or another. Music, for example, moves us physically; we tap our feet, clap our hands, or sing along and in doing so we are helped on our way. Sometimes a painting disturbs us or challenges us. Other times a poem inspires us or moves us to tears. What place do all of these things take in our everyday lives, and particularly within the everyday lives of those who are dying? Could it simply be that they elicit a response? From the isolation and paralysis of being faced with trauma such as a terminal illness, do the creative arts offer us a foundation from which to respond and find our way back into the world? Do they provide a context where we can have the opportunity to reintegrate ourselves into life, safely and actively? These are some of the questions that we seek to ask during this book.

Another aspect of the contribution of the arts is the issue of control. DeMong's (1997) American study of recreational activities in hospices argues that recreation both allows patients to become absorbed in matters other than their terminal illness and also alleviates fears of the dying process by providing dying people with an area of their lives that they can remain in control of. Hearth (Chapter 11) particularly emphasises and demonstrates how the arts can help people feel more in control, and you can see from many of the chapters in Part II how gaining control of materials and ideas as part of the creative process is a valuable experience.

As well as examining the role of the creative arts in palliative care and sharing the experiences of using them with those coming to the end of their lives, this book also offers some practical guidance for artists working in palliative care units and also for managers of those units who wish to begin to use the arts as part of what they offer. Some of the chapters that make up the second part of this book offer some useful information about activities and projects where interested practitioners may make a start, and we suggest some further reading and helpful websites that will offer further ideas at the end of each chapter. We have also supplied a list of useful suppliers at the end of the book. There is a wealth of ideas for easily achievable creative projects that will help any hospices arts service, whatever the size of the resource and, during the first part of the book, you will find some commentary and guidance on funding arts projects and employing and managing artists. However, we do not claim to provide a 'how to do it' manual. By sharing our practice and knowledge, we hope to show what might be possible on which you can build in your particular setting.

Objectives of palliative care creative arts

So far, we have been examining the range of possibilities that the creative arts offer palliative care. However, any service has to set clear objectives for its work, to establish the role of a particular area of practice within the whole and to define the achievements that it expects from its practitioners. It is often unclear whether participating in creative work is regarded either as integral to a good quality of life or as an instrument of other social objectives, such as personal growth or a sense of achievement and control of life experiences.

Some accounts of creative work in hospices, particularly Shaw's (1999) discussion, refer more clearly to its inherently valuable role as part of human experience. Thus, a good quality of life would include artistic and creative experiences, and the implication of much discussion in the literature is that this is less available for patients because of their social isolation, and because symptoms and treatment may reduce their energy and capacity to benefit from artistic experience. Therefore, it is appropriate to provide these opportunities specially, in ways relevant to their situation. In particular, people may gain continued social valuation from families and carers if they are enabled to create 'mementoes' or products. To demonstrate a social contribution to families in this way may partly respond to the wish to mimic 'work' in the daytime, to achieve outcomes or to be seen to be usefully occupied. Alternatively, activities are recognised as a good basis for facilitating social interaction and therapeutic discussion, and creative work may contribute in this way. Finally, the creative arts may ease relationships and management of the other provisions in a palliative care service.

Research and commentary on palliative day care have identified a number of issues that are also relevant to creative arts provision:

- Some analyses of objectives distinguish between therapeutic uses and leisure and supportive uses of interventions. In this book, we distinguish between the arts therapies and arts facilitation.

- Emotional, spiritual and social care objectives are rarely discussed and are not distinguished from one another; it seems that it is emotional care if it is provided by a psychologist, spiritual care by a chaplain and social care by a social worker. However, all professionals provide elements of all of these types of care, and it may be useful to try to distinguish what aspects of the achievements of the arts in each of these areas might be.

- The main aspects of interpersonal social care discussed in the day care literature refer to services that reduce isolation and increase social interactions. The creative arts may be a private and personal activity, and it is the product that may enhance social interaction, by enabling a patient to make a gift as part of a social exchange in situations where they have very little to offer others because of their illness and isolation. Undertaking arts work in a group, or participating in a group experience, may be a better means of decreasing patients' experience of social isolation. In many parts of this book, therefore, we have emphasised how groupwork may be enhanced and how joint projects may be developed.

- Experiencing arts activities at home, in a community setting or in day care also provides people with a reassuring introduction to palliative care that may make them more willing to use the services available; many people are anxious about palliative care, seeing it as 'God's waiting room'.

- Social interactions and creative work permits patients to rehearse their personal reactions to their illness and impending death in a protected and sympathetic environment with others sharing similar experiences.

- Creative work, its exhibition and its products may provide a medium for integrating family and carers into the experiences of the patient in palliative care and informing them about what is going on in the service and in the patient's emotional life.

- Creative work may offer respite for carers; Butchers (Chapter 8) gives an example of how creative work engaged a patient, enabling his wife to escape from the confines of the patient's hospice room. For many patients who are very dependent on one carer's assistance for many aspects of life, the opportunity to do something personal and separate can be useful.

Many of these objectives arise from the groupwork experience that some creative arts opportunities offer, as well as the benefits of involvement in the arts themselves. The social is in many respects indivisible from the artistic.

Creative arts as communication

Many of the chapters in this book emphasise the value of creative arts as a way of enabling communication among patients, between patients and professionals and between patients and their families and social networks. For people who are not very good with words, music or art may offer alternative forms of communication. Moreover, death and dying and the feelings that arise from patients' experience of them are difficult to convey in words. Patients may not be accustomed to the language of spiritual or reflective thought; they may not be able to analyse feelings. The creative arts may help them to express these ideas.

Just as importantly, being creative releases meaning. We start on a piece of music, art or craft and meaning emerges for us. The experience of the feel of clay, for example, may connect people with ideas in their minds that have yet to surface.

In particular, creative arts may be a way of helping palliative care services respond to diversity in the communities that they serve. This is partly because the arts are a means of communication that offers an alternative to language. Some people's language limitations may be because they come from different ethnic or language groups, or because of disabilities. Several case examples in Chapters 7–14 describe how music or art help people communicate when they have mental impairment, dementia or speaking difficulties. The arts may also help people with learning disabilities convey their experiences.

More creatively, the arts can help people express their cultural norms, cultural difference and cultural worldview. One African Caribbean woman in an art group said: 'I'm going to choose bright colours for this picture to remind me of nature back home.' Art, craft and music can help people express spiritual ideas, metaphors and preferences in ways that reflect different cultural traditions, and expand the arts in society.

A model of arts provision

Although palliative care has long used the arts as a mechanism to support its users, whether by employing paid professionals or using volunteers to provide services, it is only since the mid-1990s that there has been a real surge in the employment of artists to work as part of the palliative care team. This has been due in part to the regulation and registration as allied health professionals of arts workers such as music therapists, art therapists and dramatherapists to practise in healthcare. However, arts therapists make up only a small percentage of artists who work in hospices. During 2006/2007, the St Christopher's education centre hosted a number of days for artists working in palliative care to come together and share their work. Three groups of artists met together:

- arts therapists
- community artists and
- other arts practitioners with a range of titles, including arts facilitators, creative therapists, diversional therapists and art teachers.

They highlighted the following key themes as being important, and we have used these points as an agenda for this book:

- the need to understand and clarify the differences and similarities between arts therapists, community artists and other artists
- the problems caused by professional 'titles'
- the need for effective support and supervision

- the difficulties in articulating what artists do, and why it is important both to users and members of the multi-professional team

- the need to engage in research of the arts as used in palliative care settings and to develop suitable new paradigms.

One useful conception that emerged from the artists' meetings was the formulation of a simple model to show how the arts impact on the patients we work with, their families and carers, the organisation, the local community and the world at large. Although, during their everyday work, most of the artists focused heavily on working with patients, the model highlights the important impact that the artwork has beyond that relationship.

This concentric model allows artists to focus both inwards and outwards from their organisation. They work directly with the patient and the patient's family, but through this work also have impact on the local community and organisations within it, such as care homes, community centres and surgeries. The concentric nature of the model shows how, during the process of dying, family, community and the palliative care organisation are focusing on the patient and their needs. This does not mean that we should forget the wider influence of work with the patient, for example on the family's strength to deal with crises in the future, and on the community's awareness and valuation of the arts. The processes are also not always concentric; the patient, family and community interact independently outside the relationship with the artist and the palliative care organisation.

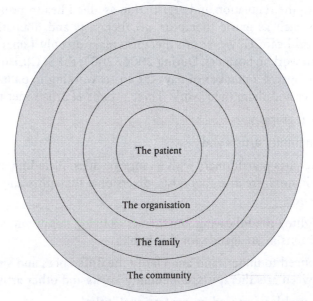

Figure 1.1 Model of the impact of arts work on patients

The patient and family also influence the palliative care organisation. The artwork begins with having impact on the patient and those immediately around them. The patient then influences others who use the organisation, either by their mood or by the artwork being exhibited within the hospice. Exhibiting has a huge influence on the environment and how users then experience it; it may brighten or stimulate the hospice or care environment, and be the catalyst for new relationships and interactions. The patient's family are also affected by the artwork, particularly if the patient gives it to them. A community exhibition of artwork will then affect the life of the community within which it is exhibited, and then through changing perceptions of those who witness the artwork exhibited, the world these people live in can be changed too. This simple model demonstrates the extent of how art created by a dying person in a hospice can affect and change the world around them, displaying the true value and meaning of the arts when used in this way.

With the growth in employment of artists in palliative care in the United Kingdom over the past ten years, we have also seen a small number of publications about the work. The music therapist Colin Lee's single case study book (1996) of working with a musician living with AIDS was one of the first publications to include a compact disc recording of the music created between therapist and patient. Camilla Connell's book on the use of art therapy in palliative care (1994) contains over one hundred art images created by people coming to the end of their lives. We are reminded here that writing about the arts is not the same as doing them, and both Connell and Lee offer the reader the possibility of witnessing what has been created alongside the written accounts of their work. We also begin to see a limited number of inquiries into the arts in palliative care settings and these are examined and expanded upon within Chapter 5 of this book. Higginson *et al.* (2000) examine the role of the arts as part of palliative care day care provision arguing that 'creative' might be a better term for Spencer and Daniels' (1998) social model of day care. Kennett (2002) highlights the place of creative arts group work within a hospice day care setting as an enhancement to emotional stability, personal enrichment and self-fulfilment. Although offering some useful insights into the arts, most of the existing research studies focus on the arts as used within specific settings and, as such, outcomes are limited. One of the strengths of the arts is that they are transferable, and are not limited by context. Music, painting and poetry, for example, can be used with people wherever they are: in their homes, in hospitals, in community centres, in their beds, wherever that bed happens to be. Future research may well need to be focused upon the expansiveness of the arts as opposed to the limitations of contexts. This expansiveness might link directly to, and support effectively, the challenges facing the development of future palliative care services at the current time in terms of exclusivity, diversity and equity.

Conclusion

This book endeavours to understand and value the place of the arts when used as part of end-of-life care. We cannot yet claim that the arts are a vital force in the future of people's care when they come to die, but we can keep the arts central within the current dialogue and debate of what will constitute an holistic, efficient and cost effective package of palliative care services for the future.

2 Managing Creative Arts and Artists in Healthcare Settings

Nigel Hartley

This chapter seeks to examine both the risks and rewards of employing and managing artists within specialist palliative care. St Christopher's Hospice is unusual in that, at the present time, we have been fortunate enough to benefit from a number of successful funding bids in order to employ a range of artists to work as part of our organisation. Many palliative care services will not be in the same position as St Christopher's and may only employ a limited arts service or volunteer help to provide artistic experiences, but the issues that arise in managing a creative arts service in palliative care are similar whatever the resources used. In this chapter, therefore, I begin by examining a range of possibilities that may be open to provide a creative arts service in a palliative care setting. I do this by describing the service provided by the different kinds of artists who work at St Christopher's, focusing on how it is managed and why. Following a personal reflection, I will then move on to look at who might best manage artists within such settings, how artists and teams of artists might be managed successfully, and how best to place them within the organisational managerial structure. I will then suggest that arts services can only be managed and developed successfully when the manager has a clear overall conception of the benefits of the arts and how they might be used as well as considering the strategic direction of the organisation and how the arts might support it. The chapter will finish with a case study of managing artists through the development and delivery of a new project within a changing environment and culture.

I do not claim that St Christopher's can show other organisations how to do it. However, by highlighting and examining what we have learned and continue to learn from our experiences of employing and working with artists, I aim to provide some insight into the options and choices that might be available for other organisations at this particular time in their development.

The St Christopher's arts service

At the present time, St Christopher's Hospice employs between 12 and 15 part-time artists. They fall into three main categories based on qualification, regulation and experience; namely, arts therapists, community artists and arts facilitators. With this staffing commitment, it is safe to assume that as an organisation St Christopher's believes that artists from each of these groups are important in bringing a range of experiences to those patients and carers under our care. A brief description of each group is as follows.

Arts therapists

Arts therapists are, at present, the only group of artists who are recognised as a profession to practise within healthcare. Over ten years ago, music therapy, dramatherapy and art therapy worked together in order to become known as the 'arts therapies', one of the 12 allied health professions (AHPs), which are registered to practise with the Health Professions Council (HPC). Therefore, with this staff group, issues of regulation and qualification are straightforward and when we employ an arts therapist the HPC provides guidance and information about things such as salary structures, what realistically to expect from a practitioner, and the need for support and supervision. Arts therapists will have gained a postgraduate qualification, during which they will have learned how to use the arts creatively within a psychological, psychotherapeutic or other disciplinary framework. They will be able to work with patients on a one-to-one basis and also with groups of patients. However, it is important to realise that the context of sessions with patients, the process of sessions with patients and the timing and regularity of sessions with patients will be key to their work; we can see this from Chapter 9 of this book. Although such therapists are able to work within a therapeutic framework, it is not unrealistic to expect them to offer other artistic experiences within the workplace such as setting up an organisational choir, organising live music events or performing live music themselves.

Community artists

Although the title 'community artist' is not protected in any formal way, a growing number of training courses have appeared in the United Kingdom over the past 10–15 years. Most of these courses will have equipped talented artists such as painters, musicians and dancers to use their skills to engage different communities of people in artistic creation. Increasingly, we come across artistic installations in towns and cities that have been created by community groups such as older people, schools, faith groups, and refugees in order to establish and claim their identity as part of the places within which they live. Although training courses exist to train artists to work in this way, some artists will still call themselves community artists even though they may have not undertaken any formal training.

Arts facilitators

Arts facilitators include artists who, although skilled as artists, may not have undertaken any formal training in how to engage a range of people in artistic experience. Others may have trained as teachers, having familiarity with teaching children or adults, but with little or no experience of working with ill people within healthcare settings. Arts facilitators may be given different names within different organisations. Examples such as diversional therapists, arts group leaders, creative therapists are only some of the terms used to describe a person doing such jobs within an organisation. Although some organisations might use the title 'artist-in-residence', it is important to understand the historical difference of this from the other names used for artists in health care. 'Artists-in-residence' would normally be an artist such as a painter, sculptor or musician who is sponsored by an organisation or individual to base themselves within a specific institution. They are furnished with their own studio or other location within the organisation in which to continue their own practice, and in return they are expected to bring their 'art' to the institution through exhibitions and workshops. On the whole, such artists are rare within healthcare settings at the current time.

In many ways 'arts facilitators', as we call them at St Christopher's, can be the most complex and interesting group of artists, since, whatever their background and experience, most of them will require a different level of training and support when entering the healthcare environment. For example, they will need to feel comfortable around ill people, understand a patient's hierarchy of needs and their own place within it, as well as finding a language in order to talk about what they do which will make sense to the wider multi-professional team.

We are more likely to come across this type of artist, whatever their job title, working within specialist palliative care units than any of the other artist groups. Among the reasons for this is the fact that many of these jobs will have grown out of volunteers providing group activities within day care settings. They will then have moved into paid employment at some stage. It is not normally as costly to employ an arts facilitator as it is to employ one of the more recognised art professions such as arts therapists, which may be an important reason why palliative care services might opt for this kind of artist.

What do artists bring to palliative care services?

At best, artists can bring a motivational energy and a positive experience both to patients who use a palliative care service and also to the service itself. Through offering patients a new experience of themselves at a time when they are dying, artists have the skill to change the nature of people's illness experience. Also, through introducing art and providing live music within the everyday fabric of the organisation, they can have a dynamic effect on the working environment in the palliative care service.

However, artists – those who bring the arts into healthcare organisations – are motivated to work in these settings for a number of reasons. As a background, they will normally have moved through school being noticed because of a particular talent within a certain art form. Studying music, they may have shown promise through performance on a musical instrument, or in an art class they may have demonstrated a skill for painting or sculpting. Whatever the experience at school, their interest or skill in music or art would have got them noticed, both actively and personally. The arts in education can be an intensely competitive place and students are told that they are 'better than' or 'more talented than' their contemporaries. This competitive bandwagon can be a damaging one. This is especially because the percentage of musicians or artists who eventually make a successful career within their particular field is small, and the effort and energy that most people put into personal development as an artist over a number of years can feel misplaced or even wasted. The majority of people who set out to develop their artistic skill as a profession will normally, following the end of a college degree, find themselves re-training in another profession in order to get a job. Alternatively, they may train as music or art teachers in order to develop the artistic skills of children for the future; the cycle will continue.

In the past, it has been rare to find a young artist moving through education who will have their sights set on bringing their art form to people who are ill. However, the emergence and development of the arts over the past 20 years as something that can benefit people's health does begin to provide another option for many artists who find themselves searching for a professional future after coming to the end of a college degree and realising that possibilities for future employment in the arts are limited. To work successfully with ill people within healthcare services, though, musicians and artists need to focus on and begin to understand their own relationship with the art forms they might use before engaging on a process of working with such people in healthcare settings.

A personal story

At this point, I would like to use my own story as an example. In many ways, it is a typical narrative of how someone might find their way to working as a musician within a healthcare setting. I began to learn to play the piano when I was four years old and remember right from the start being told that I was talented both by teachers and by my family. I moved through school devoting a huge amount of time to practice, taking all the required exams and entering music competitions. I did very well in the piano exams and won first prize in many of the competitions that I entered. I remember feeling that my career and life were mapped out in front of me and I continued developing my skill as a pianist through college. After finishing a Master's degree in performance at the age of 22, I entered the professional music circuit. Coming out of the relatively small world of college, I was shocked that the bigger professional world was confusing and complex. There were hundreds of us all competing for a tiny number of opportunities, which seemed impossible to connect with. The majority of my time was spent teaching children in order to make a living, while performing concerts when they came up, normally in small community venues on pianos that were rarely in tune. I gave up quickly, as life was limiting and depressing.

Thrown into crisis, I found myself seeing a psychotherapist to make sense of what was happening. After a time, I began to do some counselling training myself and in my mid-twenties trained as a music therapist in London. During this time, even though I was a skilled and highly trained pianist, I had great difficulty in calling myself a musician. To me, musicians were people who had made it to the top of the profession, performing and making a living from their craft. It became clear to me that, during my music therapy training using music to make relationships with damaged and sick people, I had the opportunity to put my own relationship with music right – to understand it more fully and experience the properties and dynamics of my art form in a surprising and new way. I continued to work on putting my own relationship with music right during my early years of working as a music therapist with people coming to the end of their lives, and I believe that this opportunity was vital in enabling me to work successfully over the following years.

Why tell this story? The reason is that maybe some artists who are drawn to work in healthcare settings may not have had the opportunities to begin to understand their own relationship with the arts, and this will get in the way of their art form being used in a helpful way with patients. My experience through having been involved with the training of artists to work in healthcare is that this is true of many artists beginning to work in this field. Often, managers from palliative care services contact me to say that they have employed an artist, but it has been a negative experience: patients seem not to want to engage with the arts and the artist is inflexible and is difficult to manage. Just because someone is an artist and has an interest in working in a palliative care service does not mean that they will be capable of doing it, and much thought and planning must be given when employing such people to work within such organisations. I also tell this story because, in order to manage artists successfully within a healthcare environment, it is vital to understand both an artist's background and motivation for doing this work. As using the arts in palliative care services can bring artists into close relationship with vulnerable people, it is important for the manager to pay attention to and be able to address issues as they arise, for example on occasions when an artist's personal story is getting in the way of those relationships.

One person who was employed to work as an art facilitator in a palliative care service had trained and worked as a teacher after finishing art college. A painting group was set up at the palliative care service and many patients were interested in experiencing the session. It became clear very quickly that the art facilitator expected a very high standard of painting from members of the group, and if he felt the patients' finished product was lacking in quality, he would paint over it himself so that it reached his own high standards. His actions made the patients feel as if they were constantly failing and that the art facilitator was the expert whereas, in reality, it was the artist who was failing. The manager of the service, during supervision, was able to work with the artist to realise the consequences of his actions. The artist ceased to work at the palliative care service, and this experience may have helped him explore his own relationship with his art before embarking on such work in the future.

The arts bring out strong reactions in all of us, and it is important we understand these reactions if we are to work as part of healthcare organisations that employ artists. Sometimes the work that patients produce can be intensely disturbing to us, but we cannot ask them not to paint that painting or play that music. As artists, we make the promise to accept whatever the patient produces, unconditionally and without judgement.

In addition, every member of staff who works in a palliative care service will have strong feelings about and reactions to the arts. Doctors and nurses, for example, might respond and react strongly to artists and to what they bring into the workplace. It maybe that someone reacts negatively to an artist who comes to work as part of their team because of their own relationship with the arts in the past. One nurse who sat in as part of a music group with patients kept interrupting as she wanted everyone to listen to her playing a recorder, which she had learned to play as a child. One doctor asked for an exhibition of patients' art to be removed from the hospice walls because he found it disturbing and he was afraid that other people coming through the building would be offended by the content. Most people are nevertheless moved by what they witness and are able to relate to it from their own perspective and experience.

These examples suggest that what artists bring to organisations can be complex. However, in comparison to this, they can also bring a startling simplicity and a motivational energy. Marcel (1995, p.139) captures the essence of a creative personality:

> A really alive person is not merely someone who has a taste for life, but someone who spreads taste, showering, as it were, around him; and a person who is really alive in this

way has, quite apart from any tangible achievement of his, something essentially creative about him…

The case study that concludes this chapter bears testament to this. When an organisation commits to the arts as being an important part of what it offers and stands for, the person responsible for managing artists and what they do within that organisation will also need to manage the responses and reactions of everyone who uses that organisation on a daily basis. It can be a difficult task managing such complexities.

Managing the arts within palliative care services

Most palliative care services initially introduce the arts as part of the day care services. For instance, a day centre that works with a small number of patients a day might want to find something for them to do together as a group. It may be that something is needed to negate boredom, or offer a place where patients can have a new experience by learning a new skill. Activities within day care settings are normally guided by the manager of that service and in a lot of palliative care services, they are provided by a volunteer who might have a specific interest or skill that can be applied to offer some activity or entertainment for patients.

Volunteers and professional staff

The appropriateness and role of volunteers within professional services in palliative care is a topic of current debate. There are two areas of contention. One is identifying an appropriate role for volunteers within a primarily professional service. The other is managing attitudes in a professional area where professional identity and standing are still being developed.

Recruitment and management of volunteers may be undertaken through a volunteer service supplying what is in effect a personnel support to different aspects of a palliative care service's work, or primarily through involvement in the departments providing various services. Generally, a balance between these two alternatives will be needed. The advantage of a central volunteer service is that it demonstrates to the local community, in particular volunteering organisations, a commitment to involving volunteers in the service's work. Commitment to volunteering may well be a social and political expectation from funders and commissioners of a voluntary sector palliative care organisation. A central service also operates on a time scale that responds to volunteers' needs as they are recruited and deals with issues of concern in relation to all volunteers. It is more cost-effective in providing for shared training needs than individual support and induction being provided by service managers, who have many other pressures on their time. It makes it easier for volunteers to develop a career within the palliative care organisation, meeting their changing needs and interests over the years. For example, people can start in a more routine role and with experience and training move towards counselling or personal support roles.

The advantage of service-based volunteering is that particular kinds of work may engage the interest and commitment of particular volunteers, who do not want to be bothered with wider aspects of the organisation. Nevertheless, it is important that volunteers have some understanding of and commitment to the range and objectives of the overall palliative care service. Arts work may particularly attract volunteers specifically interested in it, where volunteers with artistic skills, competence and experience may make a beeline for projects that interest them. This can bring useful resources into an arts team, particularly where resources only permit a service to employ a limited range of artists. The difficulty with organising volunteering in this way is that the service manager has to relate to, supervise and support a large number of very part-time people, who constantly change as volunteers move on to other aspects of their lives. This can make it difficult to give the time, attention and personal valuation that is an important part of motivating volunteers. Therefore, a clear strategy about what is provided centrally while at the same time developing loyalty to the service is important. At St Christopher's, recruitment and general training are handled centrally, and supervision is provided in groups for volunteers by a trainer outside the staff teams, while volunteers are integrated into the service teams and given clear guidance about the limits of their responsibilities. For example, they are required to report information about patients' concerns to professional staff, and clearly have a role in assisting professional staff to deliver their service, providing a wider range of personalities and practical support to enable groups to work well than would be possible with employed staff alone.

As the arts become more professionalised within healthcare, which has been led to a large extent by the professionalisation of the arts therapies during the 1990s, asking volunteers to provide artistic interventions in healthcare settings has become more complex and problematic. Issues may arise about qualification to practise, regulation and supervision. It is important to identify clearly what the volunteer role is in each particular instance, and to support staff to clearly value, motivate and develop the skills of the volunteers that they work with. It is easy for volunteers to feel put down by the concern of staff still finding and building a professional identity to maintain professional responsibilities. A useful resource is the guidelines published by Volunteering England about the interaction and roles of paid and unpaid staff in a variety of settings (please see the list of websites at the end of this chapter). Volunteers, who may or may not be skilled in using the arts with patients, may face barriers such as lack of access to multi-professional team meetings, patient information and records, and their very part-time attendance within the workplace. All these may be contributing factors to the complexity of integrating such services into patient care plans and the strategic direction of the organisation. It may be helpful to ensure that arts staff take the responsibility for providing adequate information to volunteers so that they can take on their role effectively with patients and feedback information that will help the staff do their job better.

The role of creative arts and artists

Also, if the arts are to be taken seriously in healthcare, integration into the multi-professional team, finding a language to describe artistic experience and developing audit and evaluation procedures should all be essential elements of current and future developments. These developments need to be spearheaded by managers of creative arts services.

In employing the three categories of arts therapists, community artists and art facilitators, St Christopher's implies a recognition of the role of artists from each of these groups. There is also an implication that each can bring equally valid contributions to St Christopher's and the patient and carer population we serve. That is, to use the arts as a psychological, therapeutic process is important for some of our users, as is giving them a less intense experience of the arts as activity. We also believe that the arts bring an important dynamic into play in relation to the different community groups around us, and how we work in partnership with them. However, there is still a lot of work needed to be done in enabling palliative care service staff to recognise the differences that each of these categories of arts work may offer. Some staff may find it hard to understand the differences between an art therapy group and a painting activity session. This can lead not only to confusion and disappointment among staff but also among patients who might attend such sessions.

As there is such a large team of artists working at St Christopher's, it has been appropriate to view them and manage them as a team, such as one might manage a team of nurses or social workers. On the most basic level, this means that the 'arts team' need their own administration space and contact facility with an appropriate level of administrative support. On another level, they meet regularly as a group, are offered individual managerial supervision and are linked into the support structures of the organisation. As with other professional groups, the arts are highlighted as a part of St Christopher's future strategic development.

In many ways, there is no difference between managing a team of artists and managing a team of doctors. Developing and understanding clear team aims and objectives and how the team relates both to the organisation as a whole and the other teams working within it are paramount. Apart from the benefits that a team of artists working together within a healthcare institution can bring, some of which are highlighted within the other chapters within this book, one major benefit has been quite surprising. If an organisation employs one or two artists to work with users, they normally belong to a day centre or a social work team, and feel that they are owned by that team and work within that team's remit. It can be difficult to develop the arts outside that remit. As a larger autonomous group, the arts team is owned by the organisation as a whole and is able to be engaged in the organisation's work in many different ways as the manager of the team and the wider organisation chooses, just as any other professional group would be. However, despite this, there are definite issues and complexities that become evident when managing any specific professions that need to be understood and related to. As a manager, grasping and understanding these issues and complexities will be vital to achieve team and organisational success.

Regular team meetings are important for any group of people working together in healthcare. Providing an opportunity to come together and learn about each other, they also provide a possibility to meet together as a group with the manager. One of the major issues for discussion during arts team meetings at St Christopher's has been that of identifying the similarities and differences between what each group of artists bring and how they work. For example, an arts therapist will place issues that are raised within a session with patients within a psychological or psychotherapeutic framework and focus heavily on the 'process' of what is created. An arts facilitator might focus completely on the quality of what is produced and, although there will have been a process, might not refer to it in the same way. Therefore, is the therapist more of an artist than the facilitator? Through dialogue and debate around such issues, we realise that although clear differences and expectations emerge there are also grey areas. We have been able to further explore these grey areas by setting up experiments when an arts therapist and an arts facilitator might run a group together. We have explored questions such as how they might support, and what they might learn from, each other in order to provide what is best for the people using the group. This debate is a continuous one, not only for St Christopher's, but also for the arts in health movement across the country. We need to continue to ask ourselves why there is a need to segregate artists into different groups within healthcare, especially at a time when there is a growing need to prove the efficacy of the arts in this area. It might be easier to create a generic role for artists within healthcare who would be able to cover all areas of need. At least then everyone might learn to know where they stand.

The team meeting also provides an important space for the manager to engage the team with understanding the strategic direction of the organisation. Major issues facing specialist palliative care at the current time, such as equality of access, the extension of quality palliative care to those living with end-of-life non-malignant disease, and the responsibility to change the experience of dying for our elderly population are only some of the topics that the arts might be able to support. During one arts team meeting, we decided to approach a number of local care homes in order to offer them some arts therapies sessions for their residents who were coming to the end of their life. Some artists were worried that if we 'watered down' what was available to patients attending the hospice building, we would be failing them. It was a difficult discussion, but we decided that people attending the hospice building would still have access to a range of support and this would not be available to those people who could not get to the building due to being housebound within a care home. A number of group sessions were offered successfully. A number of care homes have now found funding to continue to buy such sessions from the hospice. This money is used to support the arts team financially to expand and develop their work.

Individual managerial supervision sessions can also be important for artists working in palliative care services, and the reasons are really no different to any other person working as part of the team. However, due to its nature, an artist's work might be more visible within the workplace than that of most other people working there, and issues may need to be addressed and managed within individual meetings with the manager. Guidance and support for artists to help them work their way through new projects and explore innovative and fresh ways of working might be best given one to one than in a team meeting, and the opportunity for practitioners to voice more personal concerns and explore both their own limitations and their own potential should regularly be available. When art exhibitions of professional artists are successful, the artist will receive a lot of attention both from the general public and from the press. It might be important for artists working in healthcare settings to realise that it is the patients who are the artists of the work being exhibited and as such, the attention given to successful work should be focused on the patient and not the artist who worked with them. Although praise and encouragement to the artist must be an integral part of a managerial role, once again we must avoid slipping into an artist's inbuilt personal relationship with the arts. Exhibitions of patients' work must not be an opportunity for the artists who have worked with the patients to live out their own dream of being successful.

Personal support for artists working with those people coming to the end of life is needed in much the same way as any other healthcare professional working in such an environment. Structures for offering support need be built into the working day. Support happens on different levels, both formal and informal. For most staff, telling someone else what has happened enables them to move on; it is simple and straightforward. For others, a more formal support meeting might provide an opportunity to explore the affects of working with certain patients in a more detailed way. There is still much to understand about using the arts in healthcare, what they offer to people and how people are affected by arts experiences when using them in such an intense setting on a day-to-day basis. It is not usual yet to find anyone who has spent an entire career working as an artist with ill people as it is still such a new discipline. In the meantime, a range of support opportunities need to be available.

Who should manage artists working in healthcare settings?

Within any specialist palliative care institution, you come across a broad range of professional disciplines. We expect to see medical and nursing practitioners, and alongside them other professions such as social workers and chaplains.

Although within the last 20 years artists have been included within the palliative care service workforce as contributors to particular aspects of a palliative care service's work, it is still quite rare to find artists who are employed to work as part of a multi-professional team. This means that due to the part-time nature of their work, attending team meetings and making a direct input into the care plans of the patients is not seen as a priority. So, on the whole, the arts remain peripheral to patients' care and as a diversion to their illness, rather than being seen to have aims and objectives and contribute directly to their well-being. Also, if artists are employed to work in palliative care services the managerial structure under which they practise is different in each organisation.

The emergence of arts work in day care within many palliative care services, as at St Christopher's, has often been a result of the manager of day provision, although not an artist, having a strong belief in the use of the arts within such settings. Over the past four years at St Christopher's, the artists who run these groups have been joined by a range of arts therapists and a group of community artists. A separate arts team has been created in order to offer our users different artistic experiences available to them in whatever place they need them. Artists now work in a variety of community settings such as in the patient's own home, care homes and GP surgeries. When I moved into the role of managing the day unit service at St Christopher's as an artist with a long experience of working in healthcare, it seemed natural to look to expanding the arts possibilities for patients as an important thrust in the development of day services as part of the strategic direction of the organisation. My past experience as an artist made the development of a range of arts provision easier to achieve. This was helped by both an understanding of what an organisation will want and need from an artist and also what an artist will need in order to work effectively within an organisation.

It has also been important to be aware of the strategic direction of the organisation as a whole and to be both affected by it and influential within it. For example, the national drive to provide more effective specialist palliative care within an increasing number of community settings can be dramatically supported through using the arts. Picking up this strategic direction, we experimented with using the arts within different community settings, such as primary schools and care homes, in order to change the nature and experience of death within that community. Providing some group art and music sessions to residents coming to the end of their life in local care homes has had a number of effects. It has shown a group of artists that the work and responsibility of the palliative care service is much broader than just care in a specialist healthcare building. For care home nurses, seeing residents actively participating in such creative ways has changed their perception of the people for whom they are caring. As care homes witness the value of such groupwork and buy arts sessions from St Christopher's, the arts resource can be expanded and offered to other care homes who follow and gain confidence from the example of the pioneers.

An artist managing a team of artists within a palliative care service is unique and although this may provide a successful management model, it will not be possible for most organisations. There will be many different opinions regarding where the arts should sit within an organisational management structure, and it is common that artists working in healthcare settings are managed by professionals such as nurses, occupational therapists, social workers and chaplains. The decision on who manages them is a key strategic move, colouring how artists and the arts are viewed both within and outside of the organisation. Artists themselves may have the constraints of working as part of, and being managed by a manager from, another professional group. Even where there are enough artists working within an organisation to form a specific arts team, the generic professional group of the person responsible for managing and developing the arts within an institution can determine what might or might not be possible. For example, a nurse managing an artist may be protective of very sick patients by feeling that they are too ill to benefit from artistic intervention, or a social work manager may influence an arts practitioner by focusing heavily on the social and therapeutic benefits of the creative arts. Also, because of their own experiences of the arts during their lives, such professionals may have narrow or unrealistic perceptions of what is possible. Therefore, managers of such services need not only to have an interest in the arts and develop an expansive and flexible view of how they can be used, but also, like artists themselves, to have an understanding of their own relationships with the arts, what the arts can bring to an organisation and, in particular, what the arts can do for people when they are facing the end of life.

Students on placement

There are a growing number of postgraduate courses for artists to develop their skills in order to work in healthcare. The HPC and the UK Council for Psychotherapy (UKCP) are increasingly recognising arts courses as providing a valid qualification to practise within healthcare settings. Experience whilst training – 'on the job' 'in the workplace' – is vital if artists are to gain sufficient experience to work in such settings. However, the professional development of students on placement will not be enhanced if they are treated as a 'cheap option', and the possibilities for a palliative care service to provide artistic experiences are offered without committing financial and other resources to future developments. While students can provide an opportunity to test how arts might contribute, this should be part of developing a strategic vision of the role of creative arts in a palliative care service. An analogy might be made between 'using' volunteers and 'using' students to provide creative arts services without thinking through the appropriate support and development of personnel and the need for effective professional guidance in managing the service to patients.

A vital element of being a student on placement within a palliative care service is to benefit from a range of experiences such as:

- using their art form to engage with patients
- understanding how their craft – by which is meant the 'stuff' which makes up an artist's skill set, i.e. for a musician, rhythm, melody, harmony etc. or for a painter, colour, structure etc. – fits within the organisational culture
- working alongside a range of healthcare professionals
- developing a language to talk about what they do, and experience of hearing other professionals talk about what they do
- receiving informed supervision and support within the workplace.

Effective and regular supervision is vital if a student on placement is to learn from their experiences. Once more in palliative care services, we find arts students supervised by a plethora of professionals, including nurses, social workers and volunteer coordinators. In many ways, a student's role is to challenge. One of the major advantages of being a student is that they do not need to know everything. They can ask questions, challenge practice and try out things in a way that they will not be able to once they become employed practitioners. Yet again, this raises the question of who is a suitable professional person within an organisation to supervise arts students. The person needs to understand the arts and their own relationship with them, whilst encouraging and supporting the student to try new things in a safe way with the groups or people with whom they are working. The supervisor needs to work with the student on developing and claiming an authority that will be vital for their work if they are to survive as practitioners within a healthcare environment in the future. Students on placement are therefore, not a 'cheap option', but need helpful support and intervention from someone who knows what they are doing.

Arts students on placement can bring something very important into healthcare: a fresh and creative attitude, an inquiring mind and a curiosity which, if supported effectively, can be beneficial to both parties. However, when students are not given the seriousness they deserve through useful support and supervision, a placement experience can be disastrous, creating a tension and defensiveness which can be equally as damaging.

Case study

In recent years, both public education and health promotion have become a vital responsibility of many areas of healthcare. Promoting healthier attitudes to living is something we read and hear about on a daily basis. Although the hospice movement has been successful in influencing attitudes in medicine and healthcare professions towards death and dying, one of its major failings has been in changing public attitudes. For most people, although death is at some point inevitable, it is something with which they would rather not engage within everyday living. The results of a BBC poll in 2005 show that there has been little change to public attitudes towards death over the last 40 years. A current and future responsibility, therefore, must be to address this issue and work with communities of people to integrate healthily the concepts of dying and death into their everyday lives. It seems sensible, because of their expertise and experience, that palliative care services should accept his challenge.

Managing the project

As part of addressing this issue of public education at St Christopher's, one of the things we began to look at was the possibility of working with local primary schools. In Chapter 12 Sands discusses this project from the point of view of an artist involved; here I shall discuss some of the management issues and implications. Our aim was to work with children in some way: it seemed sensible, if attitudes in society as a whole were to be changed, to start with them. We were aware of the difficulties of sitting down with children in order to talk about the work of the hospice and what it did. The arts can be an indirect way of engaging with people of all ages about important issues, so it seemed apt to use them in some way when attempting to engage young children with the issues associated with the end of life.

It was absolutely vital that right from the start such a project should be supported by the palliative care service senior management team, as the danger is that such innovations might be far removed from the organisational core, and as such creates unnecessary tensions and difficulties.

Stage 1: Engaging commitment and allies and identifying barriers

The early stages of any project means engaging the commitment of the potential workforce. One major point at this initial stage was managing to get the arts team on-side, as sometimes a lack of understanding and reluctance to take part by what was to become a major part of the project's workforce can be the making or breaking of a development such as this. Therefore, it was crucial to stimulate and manage the questions and ideas that came up from the arts team. Some of the questions that came up were based around the following:

- working with children was a new experience for some of them
- the appropriateness of using the arts service in such a way
- insurance and safety
- protecting the patients
- support for the children
- parental consent

- changes in work practice and expectations
- structuring the project
- responsibilities
- use of volunteers to support the sessions.

Artists with no experience of working with children were understandably anxious about their capacity to do so, and this presented a potential practical barrier to success. Others questioned the use of our arts resource in such a way; many barriers that present themselves are strategic tensions and principles of this kind that need to be fully explored to engage commitment. It was important that the arts team should begin to understand the growing place of public education as part of a palliative care service's remit and their responsibility to respond to such challenges, and that we took the opportunity to understand their anxieties and listen to their questions. This initial stage was also important as the arts team raised some important issues that were integral to the ongoing development plan.

It is also important at an early stage to identify potential allies within the organisation, as well as colleagues who may be barriers to the success of the project, so it was a good time to look for the support of other departments. Our children's bereavement service were a vital group to have a dialogue with, both about important issues and also as to how the practitioners in that team might bring their expertise to work alongside arts team members.

Stage 2: Outreach and engagement of external partners

The second stage was to manage to make contact with a local primary school in order to gauge the responses of the head teacher and her staff to working in partnership with the hospice. We were lucky that the first school we approached were more than keen to develop both a partnership and this particular project. We met with the head teacher and the class teacher of Year Five – a group of 10/11-year-olds. Together, we decided that this would be a suitable age group to work with especially as 'loss and transition' was part of their educational curriculum. Identifying drivers and motivators that bring obvious 'wins' for potential partners can be a useful way of assuring cooperation. The group of staff who would be involved with the project also visited the hospice in order to gain a sense of the organisation, chat with some patients and also meet the artists who would be working with them. The aim of this was to develop and sustain confidence and interest in the people who could smooth any difficulties that might arise for the partners.

Stage 3: Planning the project

At this point, we decided on a project programme, since explicit planning can motivate people and raise their confidence that they can handle difficulties that might arise. The programme would run over about six weeks, including one session a week. Sessions three to six would take place within the hospice, whilst the initial two sessions would take place back at school and would include an introduction to the history of St Christopher's whilst introducing the children to its place within their community. The other four sessions would include the following:

- A visit to the school by the arts team manager and the manager of the children's bereavement service. This would include a question and answer session with the children, both to discover what the children had learned during the previous two sessions, but also to address any questions or anxieties. Following this meeting, the children would visit the hospice with their teachers. They were introduced to two artists who would work with them over the next two sessions and also to a group of patients. During this session children and patients could ask each other questions.

- Sessions four and five would include two further visits to the hospice, when the children and patients could create some large art pieces that would be exhibited back at their school. The work created would be a joint decision between the children and the patients, and they would be supported and guided by the two artists.

- The final session would be a celebration back at the hospice to which the children would invite their parents and the patients would invite any family members and friends. This would take the form of a feedback session, focusing on what has been gained and what has been learned from the experience. As well as exhibiting the artwork created, there would be an opportunity for the children to sing and recite poetry together. This celebration would conclude with a tea party during which volunteers from the hospice would provide hospitality.

The experience of the project is described by Sands in Chapter 12.

In managing such a project, it is, therefore, important that the manager is a key figure in working separately with the different groups involved, as well as being a lynchpin in bringing all parties to work together effectively. Funding and costing will be touched upon briefly in Chapter 4, which also includes an example of a simple funding application. Although artists will probably be paid anyway for their work at the hospice, the costs of things such as arts materials, travel back and forth between hospice and school, and food should be given careful consideration and should be clear to all participants to avoid disputes or losses arising unexpectedly. The manager needs to work together with the school to share such costs, where possible.

In order for such a project to develop successfully, the main points to focus on are as follows:

- understanding the organisational strategy and needs of participants in both organisations

- working with the senior management team to ensure support if difficulties arise, particularly in public perception – for example, palliative care service funders or commissioners saying that this is inappropriate work for the palliative care service to be doing, or parents questioning whether their children should be involved with this subject

- supporting and working with the artists

- working with other palliative care service departments to gain support and additional relevant resources within their priorities

- discovering an appropriate partner, in this case a school with an understanding head teacher and class teachers

- clearly defining the project's aims and objectives, avoiding misunderstandings and ensuring commitment to them from potential dissenters

- planning the project programme

- costing and funding.

Through managing such projects a lot is learned. At St Christopher's, we have now completed the 'Schools Project' with a number of different primary schools, and this number continues to grow due to demand.

Conclusion

In many ways, managing artists is no different from managing any other professional group of people, and nor should it be. However, as with any professional group, it is important to develop a deep understanding of the kinds of people who make up such a professional workforce. Among the factors that help a manager is to identify the common aspects of the development of the artists' artistic careers and experiences that they have lived through, and also the reactions and responses that both their individual and collective crafts can bring to a palliative care service, to patients, other staff and volunteers. In this way, it is possible to ensure that different kinds of artistic contribution can achieve an impact like that of other professions in playing their part within the development of organisational strategy and become integrated into the multi-professional team.

In summary, although management is management whatever the organisation, the special features and challenges of individual personalities and the collective contribution of a group of professionals to an organisation needs to be taken seriously and, consequently, valued and understood.

Further reading

Armstrong, M. (2006) *A Handbook of Human Resource Management Practice* (10th edn). London: Kogan Page.

Atrill, P. and McLaney, E. (2004) *Accounting and Finance for Non-Specialists* (4th edn). Upper Saddle River, NJ: Prentice Hall.

Johnson, G., Scholes, K. and Whittington, R. (2005) *Exploring Corporate Strategy* (7th edn). Upper Saddle River, NJ: Prentice Hall.

Mintzberg, H., Ahlstrand, B. and Lampel, J. (1998) *Strategy Safari – the Complete Guide Through the Wilds of Strategic Management.* Upper Saddle River, NJ: Prentice Hall.

Whittington, R. (2000) *What is Strategy – and Does it Matter?* (2nd edn). London: Thomson.

All these books are general management texts that will be useful for managers seeking self-development.

Websites

www.hpc-uk.org – Health Professions Council – registration body for arts therapists, accessed on 13 February 2008.

www.UKCP.org – UK Council for Psychotherapy, accessed on 13 February 2008.

3 The Palliative Care Community – Using the Arts in Different Settings

Nigel Hartley

In this chapter, I address both the complexities and benefits that come from working as an artist within different palliative care contexts. This includes an examination of the growing need for palliative care to support and provide a more comprehensive set of supportive services within a range of community settings such as the patients' own homes, care homes and GP surgeries. The chapter includes examples to highlight important issues that arise when working as part of a multi-professional team in a number of different contexts, and ends with a brief review of the arts and how they relate, or are seen to relate, to illness and health.

Hospices or specialist palliative care units have always provided services outside the physical buildings that the organisation inhabits. Inpatient units, day units or outpatient clinics offer services to only a part of the patient population that the institution serves. The majority of patients and their families will never visit the buildings from which these units work and will receive most of their care in the last months of life at home or in other places where they live such as care homes. Some people will choose not to visit the hospice or specialist palliative care unit because they do not want to, others because they are isolated by the physical and emotional aspects of their illness within their own homes and are unable to leave them.

Hospices, in particular, have championed highly effective specialist community nursing. Of course, a community nurse specialist engages with those they care for in the home well beyond the confines of pain and symptom management. They will be skilled enough to address a broad range of psychological, social and spiritual issues that their patients and carers often raise. However, this may not be enough and social workers, for example, will be expected to make home visits and in doing so address some of the more complex psychological and emotional issues that patients and carers raise. However, nurses and social workers cannot meet the needs of all patients in every situation. For example, many people coming to the end of their lives may need support in ways other than using everyday speech and language due to communication or problems with articulation. As highlighted in the second part of this book, the arts can offer a useful medium when used with such patients.

As already discussed in Chapter 2, artists are motivated to work in healthcare settings for a variety of reasons; their background, experiences, education and personality will all affect the work that they do and how the patients and carers that they encounter during that work will engage with them. Arts therapists, for instance, will come with a formal postgraduate training; they will expect to work within a specially designed therapy room and to receive referrals from the multi-professional team. Artists who are used to working in education, however, teaching people how to paint, draw or make pottery, will expect the groups of people they work with in healthcare settings to fall into much the same framework to that they are used to. Both of these examples may not entirely be what an organisation, patients or carers want from an artist.

When employing an artist, organisations may want a variety of things, but whatever the artist's qualifications or background, some or all of the following should be included:

- *To be able to engage patients and their carers in a variety of different settings.* It must be clear from the outset that the artists employed will be required to use their skills in a variety of locations, both within and outside the organisational building. This will require a flexible mix of strengths and skills.

- *To be able to articulate their work in a clear way that means something to patients and their carers and also to members of the multi-professional team; to be able to contribute to overall care plans for patients.* It is expected that artists will be able to explain to patients and their carers what is required from them when they get involved, what to expect when they do, and why the creative arts might be useful to them at this stage in their lives. They will also be required to note their interventions within patient records. Attending multi-professional team meetings and listening to and understanding the interventions of other health and social care professionals as well as being able to talk about and explain their own work in relation to the rest of the team will also be a major requirement.

- *To be able to exhibit and perform artwork in public settings.* Artists must understand both the need and the benefits of exhibiting the artwork created on the hospice or unit site and in a variety of community locations and this is discussed in more detail in Chapter 4. They will need to know how to exhibit artwork effectively and the artists will need to act as ambassadors for the organisation. They must understand how the artwork itself can be used to raise awareness of the organisation and the work that it does, whilst also using the opportunity to enable changes to occur around perceptions of death and dying within the wider community.

- *To be able to work in partnership with a variety of community groups, planning and delivering short-term arts projects.* Creating relationships with community groups, such as specialist health and social care professionals, schools, art establishments and faith centres should also be an important part of an artist's work. This will be particularly important when setting up health promotion projects and community exhibitions.

- *To be a practising artist.* Finally, but most importantly, artists working in healthcare must continue to practise their own art discipline themselves. The importance of continuing to practise their own art forms is that it will keep them in touch with the very essence of the work they are doing with patients and carers, as well as enabling them to develop new concepts and ideas which will be invaluable for their work in healthcare. For example, for a musician working in healthcare, it will be useful to keep up to date with developments within all areas of the world of music, including music from different cultures and music from a range of different musical styles such as popular or current day 'classical' music. The main reason for this is that when meeting new patients and users, they must be able to engage with them from the patients' own musical or artistic starting point. The art or music used may not be the personal preference of the artist, but it is important that this does not get in the way of the creative process.

Examples of different settings

Day care

Artists who work within day care settings must be integrated into the everyday working ethos and philosophy of the units themselves. Aims should include the possibility for patients to learn to cope more effectively within the communities in which they live the majority of their lives and to feel more secure with their illness and everyday experiences.

It is common for artists employed to work within a hospice or specialist palliative care unit to be placed within day care centres or outpatient clinics. The reasons for this will vary, but may include the fact that a group of patients already exist and it will be easier for the artist to work with them either as a group or as individuals within this context. Also, even though the artist may be employed on a part-time basis it is relatively easy for them to feel part of a team, because they will normally engage with that team for a whole day at a time. During the day, they will be able to engage in daily team meetings and feel part of the unit structure. Specialist palliative day care has grown in popularity over the past 20 or so years, but more recently, challenges posed by the publication of the NICE guidance in 2001 and a small number of research reports (Douglas *et al.* 2003) question the benefits, need and the appropriateness of such services. These include issues such as 'exclusion' and 'equity', which are highlighted by the number of people who access day care units representing only a small percentage of the patient population of many organisations and the cultural mix of patients attending not being a reflection of the local community population. In addition, the lack of any consensus about appropriate models of day care means that the structure of each day care unit differs greatly from the next and the range of services offered in one unit may bear little resemblance to those offered in another unit. Patients who attend day care units often require a complex mix of care and support. There will certainly be pain and symptom management, best delivered by a specialist medical and nursing team. However, the fact that these people have been referred into a context that brings a number of people in a similar situation together needs to be addressed. Patients are accessing a large part of their specialist care within this specific context. It is likely that these people will have social issues, which need to be addressed such as isolation due to difficult family dynamics or a lack of informal care within the place that they live. Addressing complex social issues will be key if these people are to be supported in order to cope with their everyday situations more effectively outside of the day unit.

Aims, objectives and groupwork styles are therefore vital aspects to be taken into consideration when working with both groups and individuals in such settings. Much of the thinking around offering creative arts groups within hospice day units has concentrated on the arts as diversion (Kennett 2002). Many activities have the possibility to divert our attention for periods of time, and some patients facing a terminal illness and all that this brings will discover, with some help and support, how this might work for them. However, the benefits of diversion are limited, and if day units include creative arts groups within their programme, it is important that there is a common consensus as to why this is. Creative arts divert the mind to a certain extent but as a means to an end this theory sells the arts short of their most central usefulness (Hartley 2007). The arts contain within them a unique set of motivational properties and dynamics. The fact that the arts move us physiologically, psychologically and emotionally places them as important tools when dealing with common responses to a terminal illness such as depression, lack of meaning and direction, and fear of the future.

One criticism of day care units within hospices is that they create a culture of dependency for their users; that is, people come to rely on a high level of support, finding it hard to face life without it. Where day care units discharge patients, this is becoming increasingly problematic. Normally a patient will attend a day care unit for one day every week; during that day they will experience a high level of care and attention which offers them a very different reality to that of their everyday lives which are difficult for a range of reasons. If discharge from the service is to remain a possibility, then helping people discover and develop new skills and strategies to cope with everyday life more successfully must be a vital aim. There can be no point in offering people a day every week when they can escape from a problematic reality, in order to expect them to return to that reality exacerbating the problems that exist because their life feels better during that weekly visit to the day unit. Although the weekly visit can offer the patient some short-term respite from the difficulties they are encountering, it does not normally offer them the possibility of changing their ongoing problems for the better unless this aim is part of the planned agenda.

Different kinds of groupwork offer a range of experiences and possibilities, which enable people to discover new strengths and new skills in order to cope with the difficulties in their lives. The arts are not the answer to all the problems that our patients face, but used as part of a planned supportive programme they can motivate groups of people to view things differently and cope more effectively.

Some artists will offer a range of creative possibilities, using the arts to enable each person within the group to work on an individual creation; there are some examples in Part II of this book of working on individual paintings or individual craft pieces. Patients are normally pleased and surprised at what is possible, most of them creating objects of good quality that they can give to relatives or friends, or even to the organisation itself to exhibit as a mark of pride and thanks. This kind of experience within a group is useful in that it can change the perception of both the patient and those around them, from people with lives which feel as if they are disintegrating into people with lives that can be lived with more meaning and fulfilment. However, there are dangers here in terms of the possibility of isolating patients even more. In supporting individuals to work by themselves within the group we must be careful that they don't remain just that, individuals, whilst the benefits of a group experience are missed. This kind of group style can also be resource heavy; some artists who work in this way expect a high number of other staff or volunteers to support them in their work as each patient might require a high level of one-to-one support to develop their own creation. Volunteers can be a useful resource in supporting any kind of group activity, but training and education about roles and expectations within such groups must be built in to the more general training of both volunteers and artists. This has been discussed in some detail in Chapter 2. It is more likely that artists running groups in a day care setting will encounter volunteers than in any other specialist palliative care setting. It is therefore paramount that attention is given to clarifying the expectations of the artists, the volunteers and the organisation as a whole. It is also important that artists working with groups within day care settings feel confident enough to develop group aims and objectives within the arts projects that they undertake. Some day units use volunteers to deliver and facilitate art groups, as this reduces the funding demands of employing people to carry out the work. However, the staff resources required to induct, train, support and supervise volunteers to carry out such work must be taken into consideration.

Engaging creatively with the arts can generate strong reactions in some patients as powerful feelings and memories are stirred and raised. It is therefore important that creative arts groups are run not only by skilled professional artists, but by artists who have the capacity to work as part of the team and relate confidently with other professionals. Paying skilled artists also gives a message of how seriously the organisation takes this kind of work. Working as part of the day unit team is paramount if artists are to support the aims and objectives of the team as a whole. They should also be able to instil a secure group feeling by how they facilitate their work. Asking the group to begin by telling each other something that has happened to them during the week can be a useful way to create a sense of belonging. Some artists worry that asking patients how they are feeling should be left for the therapist. Asking people how they are feeling is, however, a human activity which can let the patients know that they are cared about, and give them an experience of being listened to, heard and understood.

For example, one group of patients who came to a hospice day centre were keen to create a piece of artwork that could be displayed within a new community centre within the area in which most of them lived. They discussed this with an artist who worked at the hospice and asked for guidance and support. After discussion with both the artist and the management team of the community centre, they decided to create a 12-foot square mosaic, depicting community landmarks that had been important to them in their lives. The artists worked with them to create a design that included their local pub, school and church, the hospice and the community centre itself. The design was created incorporating the doorways of all the buildings depicted and the topics of discussion during the creation of the mosaic included a number of related topics such as the symbolic meaning of a doorway, the doorways they had encountered during the lives and the doorway between life and death. As the mosaic was created by the group and the tiles were placed on the design piece by piece, memories of entering and leaving each of the institutions depicted were shared, as well as a more metaphorical discourse around the meaning of doorways, entrances and exits as mentioned above. The group worked with the artist on the mosaic during six visits over six weeks to the hospice day unit. Once it was completed, the mosaic was hung in the reception of the new community centre along with a plaque describing the story of its creation along with the names of those involved. This experience of creating together affected the lives of both patients and day centre staff during those six weeks, strengthening relationships, deepening understanding and motivating a group of people to attempt to make sense of both their living and dying. The patients in the group made a strong bond with each other and began to meet together in smaller groups outside the hospice day centre during the week, for a coffee, for lunch or just for a chat. Some, who had been relying heavily on family members and carers, showed signs of becoming more independent. Others, who lived alone, found a new community of caring to which they belonged, which existed outside of the hospice building. All of them, even if only for short periods of time, found new ways of living and of coping that were not dependent on the hospice services.

Inpatient units

Artists need to feel confident and secure with their own skills and abilities when working within inpatient settings. Patients and carers expect to see doctors and nurses within a healthcare setting, but we must remember how bizarre and unexpected it might be when someone approaches the bedside with a guitar or a set of paints. Much thought needs to be given by both the artist and the organisation to how the arts are introduced into their world and healthcare experience. Because users of inpatient units may not see artists as central to the healthcare experience, but as external or additional, perhaps not part of the healthcare contract with the institution, it is important that they are told of the full membership of the multidisciplinary team – from doctors and nurses, through to physiotherapists, occupational therapists and artists. They need to feel confident that all members of the team are skilled and compassionate professionals, each with their own place and purpose within the patient care plan. There are many ways to do this. In some circumstances, artists might approach patients and carers for the first time themselves. Often, however, an introduction from a nurse or a member of the wider team is useful. This can explain what a meeting with an artist might achieve for them. It can help to allay patients' and carers' fears, as well as acknowledging and accepting the arts as something worthwhile as part of healthcare provision. Getting explanations and introductions right can be complicated since what is right for one may not be right for others, but they are vital, since for many people at this particular time of their lives the arts will appear at once distance and strange and can remain so due to fear or lack of interest.

Within specialist palliative care inpatient settings it is likely that an artist will encounter patients who are facing the reality of the imminent end of their life or who are experiencing issues such as severe physical or psychological pain (Hartley 2005). There may also be a high level of anxiety among carers and relatives and sometimes even among members of the multi-professional team itself. Because the artist is probably working part-time, it may be more difficult for them to become part of that team within the inpatient context and they may feel isolated and unsupported when working in this particular arena. It often proves to be a difficult matter, but if organisations are committed to artists working within all possible settings, the problems that come with employing someone to work part-time within an inpatient setting need to be given some careful consideration. The artist will be used to working with groups within the day unit at pre-arranged times, but within an inpatient ward they will now find themselves in uncharted territory regarding the flexibility of time management that is needed. Working with patients and families within an inpatient context will require the artist to juggle their timing and availability with more regular commitments, and a hasty response may not be possible. Many patients within a specialist palliative care inpatient unit may spend many hours alone during the day. However, for some, a programme of individual appointments with the medical consultant, the nurse, the social worker and the physiotherapist, combined with a more flexible programme for physical and psychological support and together with visits from family or friends, generates a complex daily programme, which can be difficult to claim a part in. After a packed programme of such appointments and interventions, it may be that a patient is just not feeling energetic enough, or does not see the point of meeting with an artist. Although it may not be possible for an artist to take part in weekly ward rounds or team meetings, it is important that they take time to forge relationships with members of the inpatient team in order to become accepted and trusted. Being present at daily handover meetings will be an important way of becoming known; taking time to engage with nursing staff at appropriate times will be a useful part of the work and the artists themselves becoming accepted.

Taking the arts to the bedside can be extremely rewarding, although sometimes complex and risky. Working with a person as they lie in their bed or are within the confines of their own living space can throw up issues around what is appropriate and what is not. One example is of an elderly Greek woman who was dying in a hospice inpatient ward. She spoke hardly any English and most of her family lived abroad. One of the nurses asked if a musician might visit her, because the team felt as if they were making very little contact and that the patient appeared withdrawn and depressed. The musician visited her, and using a guitar to accompany them, they began to sing Greek folk songs together. The woman's involvement was minimal at first, but gradually she became more involved, changing from singing at key moments within the songs such as at the end of musical phrases, to initiating new songs and clapping her hands along in time to the music. The nursing team were energised by seeing an example of how one of the arts can draw someone out of isolation into a lively and dynamic relationship. Because of this, they felt less drained and frustrated in terms of caring for her. Some days later, as the patient slipped into a coma, her family arrived from Greece to be with her; they felt frustrated that they had arrived at a time when it was not possible to engage with their loved one. When the musician came to the ward again, the family were there visiting. The family's initial reaction was to protect the patient from an activity that they felt sceptical about. As the musician began to play music, the family joined in and sang familiar Greek folk songs around the bed of the dying woman; from time to time the patient tapped her hand in time to the music. Following the death, the family commented that it was during the music making that they had made the final contact with their relative; they were grateful.

The community

The hospice or specialist palliative care unit is not just a building. In most hospices, only a small percentage of the patient population will visit the hospice building during their illness, most of their care being delivered within the places that they live. The places where people live as they are dying include the homes they have lived in all of their lives, but are not restricted to these. People die in places such as hospitals, care homes, hostels and prisons, and specialist palliative care staff will need to deliver their services within a range of physical spaces within the community away from the organisations that they are employed by.

The arts have little restriction and few boundaries; they exist in all cultures and all communities, and each of us will have been touched by them during our lives. Some people will have had negative experiences at school; many of the artists writing in Part II describe patients feeling inhibited from starting to use creative arts in palliative care because of such bad experiences. Others will have physically engaged with one or more of the creative art forms during their lives by singing in a local choir, or attending a painting or writing class. People might have enjoyed the arts from a slight distance, observing exhibitions in art galleries, attending concerts or enjoying music at home. Whatever people's experiences of or attitudes towards the arts, they will carry with them strong memories, feelings and responses which will influence how they might or might not engage with the arts at the end of their lives.

Visiting and working with patients at home needs skill and sensitivity. It will be unlikely that many artists coming to work in healthcare will have experience in this area. Sometimes, the experience of visiting a patient within their own home can be both surprising and challenging. Bell (1998, p.88) tells us of such an experience when visiting a patient at home for an art theerapy session:

> passing through the living room David leaned over his father's shoulder and peering at the picture in front of him, said, in a broad Yorkshire accent, 'when tha's finished that, tha can paint the side o' my van!'…this incident was really only a taste of the unpredictable peculiarities of spending time with people in their own home…

Therefore, time must be taken to develop through training and education skills to prepare and equip them to carry out this kind of work safely and effectively. Most palliative care services have community nurse specialists who work with patients and families at home and liaise with other community professionals. It can be useful for an artist to link up with these nurses. Observing their work and spending time with them can offer possibilities for artists to learn and feel at ease within this world. Working alongside nurses is also important because it will be these people who will trust the artist's abilities and refer patients to work with them.

When entering someone's home, it could be that we are entering into the most intimate of places. This is the patient's territory, where they call the shots and control what will or will not happen. However, the home environment immediately provides the artist with a range of information regarding a person's tastes and life experiences, which can offer a practical and positive place to start. When visiting a man who presented as depressed and stuck in the home for the first time, an artist drew the patient's attention to a painting hanging above the fireplace. The painting depicted a flamenco dancer in full flight, with a group of people watching, laughing and full of energy. The patient observed the painting for some time and then told that artist that although the painting had been there for over 30 years, he had rarely looked at it in any great detail. His parents had bought it when they were still alive and he remembered them bringing it home for the first time. Now, observing it in detail he was clear that it wasn't to his taste. The man's wife, who was also present, told both her husband and the artist that she too had never liked it, but had never wanted to say so because she knew it had been bought by her husband's parents and she had not wanted to upset anyone. Together they decided that they would like to paint something to take its place. Talking with the couple, the artist learned that they had visited the Tate Modern gallery in London a number of times, and were particularly drawn to the more abstract and colourful artworks on display. Over three visits, the artist and the couple created an explosion of colours and shapes together which they named: 'The Colours of Our Life'. The painting was framed and signed and now hangs over the fireplace in the home. The wife can observe the painting, an object left behind that holds some vibrant and positive memories of both her husband and their relationship during the last weeks of his life.

A community nurse specialist asked a musician to visit an older woman who was coming to the end of her life in a care home. The lady was living alone, since her husband had died a number of years previously and her only child lived in Australia. With the musician, the lady chose to sing a range of important songs from her life, telling stories of the times when the specific songs had been important to her. They ranged from Victorian parlour songs to the songs of Cole Porter, George Gershwin and Rogers and Hart. The care home staff felt enlivened by the old lady's singing, because it introduced to them a part of her that they had never known. In between the musician's visits, they continued to sing along with her and some of the other residents joined in too. The care home manager had a sum of money in the budget to develop activities and therapeutic work. He had never used it because it was difficult to find people with suitable experience and ability to come and work with them.

The care home manager made a contract with the hospice in order to buy in music sessions for all the residents in the care home. The musician visits the home once a week and runs a music group open to everyone who lives there. The care home pays the hospice directly for the music service and the hospice agrees to supervise and support the musician and their work. This is an important agreement, showing that there are possibilities for hospice staff to work closely with community groups around them in new and creative ways, fulfilling a number of social, political and economic challenges. There has been some positive feedback from the care home staff; they believe that the weekly group brings the home and the residents to life, drawing them out of themselves positively into the world.

Art and illness

Hospices and specialist palliative care units have a responsibility to engage and work with the communities they serve. For all its success, one of the major failures of the modern hospice movement has been in strengthening the confidence of people in the communities that hospices serve to take a role in death, dying and the challenges that this brings. As we move into a new era of development for end-of-life care, working with communities to create healthier responses to death and dying will most certainly need to be a priority. Although it might seem that art and illness do not sit happily together, there is an important and productive role to be played: 'at first glance the concepts of "art" and "illness" do not seem to go together. Art and creativity are active, whereas illness seems passive…' (Kaye 1998, p.38).

The creation of any of the arts is an active process, and part of their real strength when used during illness is to motivate people to stay present in the world in a way which brings together dynamically both being and doing. Over the past ten years, a drive to introduce the creative and performing arts into more public places within health and social care settings has begun to change dramatically the nature of our experience of illness and being cared for. Creative artists and the creative arts bring an energy to an organisation, a liveliness which is not often found in the workplace today. The acts of creating art, performing music, constructing and exhibiting paintings can change environments from something commonplace into a space with interest, energy and atmosphere. An organisation that employs artists and puts the experience of creating and exhibiting artworks on the agenda for its patients, carers, staff and visitors makes a unique statement. Although experiencing the arts can change the nature of people's deaths and those around them, the fact that the arts are being created as part of everyday life both in organisations like hospices and in other community organisations can change the fabric of the organisation and the world's view of it.

Part II of this book tells stories and provides guidance for both artists working in end-of-life settings and those who manage their work. We must bear in mind, though, that writing about the arts and the creative processes is not the same as doing them. Because the arts are not based in, and indeed are often used as a replacement for everyday language, when attempting to translate them back into words something essential will be lost. During the chapters, we witness a range of different descriptions, each writer giving their unique perception of the work they do and what it means to them. Every one of us will respond differently to creating or viewing art: even though we all see or hear the same thing, both our psychological and our physiological responses will differ (Ansdell 1995). There is about the creative process and the object that is created something of the wordless; no group of words can accurately describe what is seen or heard. It is not new that artists have a responsibility to struggle to define and articulate both what they do and what it all means. However, it is many centuries since the arts have been witnessed as an important part of people's healthcare (Kearney 2000). In a modern healthcare system, at the heart of which lies a medical profession that will settle for nothing less than descriptions made with cut-glass precision and accuracy, the creative arts may seem strange bedfellows. Nevertheless, when working in such settings, artists must push ahead with continuous sustained inquiry into their work; what they are doing, which theories underpin it, and how it all works are all parts of the jigsaw if the marriage between medicine and the arts is ever to be successfully re-established:

> research, theory and practice are closely interrelated. They enrich, inspire and emerge from one another, and act in tandem to one another. Any less intimate relationship between them does no service to any of them – or to the arts…professions… (Ansdell and Pavlicevic 2001, p.21)

Further reading

Aldridge, D. (ed.) (1998) *Music Therapy in Palliative Care: New Voices.* London: Jessica Kingsley Publishers.

A comprehensive account of different models of music therapy as used within palliative care.

Bell, S. (1998) 'Art Therapy in the Community.' In M. Pratt and M. Wood (eds) *Art Therapy in Palliative Care.* London: Routledge.

A useful discussion of art therapy in community settings.

Dileo, C. and Loewy, J. (eds) (2005) *Music Therapy at the End of Life.* Cherry Hill, NJ: Jeffrey Books.

A recent account of the development of music therapy within end-of-life care.

Kennett, C. (2002) 'Psychosocial Day Care.' In J. Hearn and M. Myers (eds) *Palliative Day Care in Practice.* Oxford: Oxford University Press.

A useful general article about palliative day care practice, incorporating a strong focus on the arts.

4 Exhibiting, Promoting and Funding the Arts in Healthcare Settings

Nigel Hartley

This chapter highlights the potential for the artistic products created by patients and carers within hospice settings to be used as part of exhibitions, or as an important element within the production of organisational promotional material. It begins by asking some questions (Ansdell and Hartley 2000) based around the place of the arts within society, and then moves on to examine the differences and tensions that arise between the artistic process and the artistic product. A short section follows that highlights some important issues about funding arts projects within palliative care settings. This section includes an example of a simple funding application. The aim of the chapter is to raise some challenging questions regarding the use of the artwork created by people who are ill whilst providing a simple guide to exhibiting artwork within community settings.

Issues in exhibiting creative arts from healthcare settings

What is art for?

Most of us will observe art every day. We will also hear music, live or recorded, many times and in many different places on a daily basis. The majority of us display artwork within our own homes, as well as regularly listening to favourite recordings of music that we like. Most of the environments that we work in will be enhanced and supported by works of art in order to provide an experience of value whilst we do our jobs. Why is this so? Although many of us will find it hard to articulate the reasons why the arts play an important part in our lives, somehow we all know that art has the potential to move and inspire us, grab our attention and change who we are and most importantly the way that we relate to the world and those around us.

Although there are a few examples over the years of professional artists not wanting the work that they have created to be seen, most art, for example painting, music, dance, poetry and sculpture, is created to be witnessed. This regularly happens formally within museums, concerts halls and theatres where the artistic product is observed and responded to, but also happens informally within the places that we live and work as already mentioned. Although the expression and motivation of the artist who produces the art is central and the process of creating will have been integral to their own lives and experiences, the product created is then given over to the public who are entertained, moved, inspired or disturbed from their own personal perspective. Such responses give the artistic product value and can have an important part to play in the success of both the product and those who created it; in Chapter 2 I discussed, using my own experience, the motivation of artists to be successful producers of artistic products. However, when the arts are viewed in this way, little is known about how the work came into being, of the process involved or of the life of the artist. This kind of information is part of the literature, criticism and history of music, art and creative writing, but is not intrinsically part of the artistic product. It comes out in the exhibition or programme notes or critical literature.

When the arts are used in healthcare, we often focus on the process of creating art as being the core rationale for engaging patients within such an activity. Comparing that focus with the way in which the arts are commonly used within society, it could be seen as counter-cultural that the patient is not given the opportunity to exhibit the product created and, therefore, benefit from the responses and reactions of those around them.

How do we train artists?

Is the emphasis in the traditional training of artists right? Artists are taught techniques in order to create their work. The development of these techniques leads to artists developing preferences about how they work, what sort of work they produce and the materials they use. How well artists use certain techniques will normally be key in assessing their expertise and in how their work is viewed and critiqued. Many works of art are created in isolation. That is, one artist will absorb themselves in a process that takes place away from the bump and grind of everyday life and, therefore, away from relationships with other people. If most works of art are created in isolation, are we therefore in danger of producing artists who find it difficult to relate flexibly and confidently with other people? Should we be rethinking the way in which we train them?

The major focus in using the creative arts within healthcare settings has to be on the relationships that artists make with patients and the relationships that patients make with each other. Out of these relationships, patients discover the essence of what the arts can bring both to themselves and also to their lives during illness. For that reason, should artists working in healthcare feedback their experiences into generalist arts education, and by doing so, create the possibility to rediscover and redefine the place of both artists and the arts within society (Bunting 2007)?

What is art like?

Although each art form has its own unique properties and dynamics (Hartley 2007), is there something that binds them together in terms of both process and product? Is art an object, and do we teach artists to think of it in this way, as it is the product that may bring them fame and fortune and not the process of how it is created? For example, thinking about music, musicians study 'it' and they perform 'it', they write 'it' and they analyse 'it'. With painting, artists study 'it', create 'it', and with poetry, poets write 'it' and people read 'it'. When we witness art exhibited or music performed, 'it' is the thing we go and look at or listen to, 'it' is the thing that we relate and respond to. How do we understand the relationship between the product we witness and the process of how 'it' came into being and does this relationship matter?

The arts in health provide a context where both process and product can be equally valid, and the fact that the art is created as part of different relationships places the arts, how and why they are created, into a unique framework. Can the arts as used in healthcare therefore be instrumental in relating artistic structures and processes to human structures and processes? Rather than just producing art for commercial reasons and creating art that nobody wants to look at, can artists working in healthcare offer a new way for the arts to be viewed and valued within society?

Who is artistic?

As I discussed in Chapter 2, professional artists will at some point in their lives have been told that they are talented. Saying that some people are 'artistic' and have a talent separates them from other people who are not 'artistic' and do not have a talent. Is it only the gifted few that are artistic, those who make a profession out of it in some way?

In healthcare, as many of the authors of the chapters in Part II describe, it is common to come across patients who, when introduced to the idea of creating art, will respond negatively, saying that they are not talented or cannot do it. Such reactions may have their roots in being told during their education that they are not artistic. Sometimes this has led them to believe that they are not talented and they have distanced themselves from the act of creating art throughout their lives. Artists working in healthcare settings will begin from the premise that everyone can create something of meaning and value through the creative arts. Do they therefore challenge the exclusive attitude that the creative arts are owned only by the gifted few?

Wherever the creative arts are used, we cannot ignore the common facts and experiences of how they are created and why they are created. A successful artist creating works of art and exhibiting them within a public venue will and must engage in similar experiences to those of a person dying of cancer in a palliative care service who paints a delicate watercolour or makes a pot, which is then shown as part of a community exhibition. One of the only differences might be that no money changes hands. However, even art created by dying patients might be sold to make money, or as an opportunity to raise funds for the organisation that it represents.

Exhibiting art – promoting creative work in palliative care

At St Christopher's Hospice, it has already been mentioned that we employ a variety of artists to work with our patients. Some of them, particularly the arts therapists, will have been taught a discipline where process is the main focus, and the purpose of the product is to use it as an object for analysis between the therapist and the person who created it. Beyond this, the arts therapists will have been taught that the object is 'confidential' and it will then remain hidden away. Taking into account that in everyday life most art that is created is witnessed, critiqued, and bought, this concept of the arts being 'confidential' could be counter to most people's common experiences. Having worked as a music therapist for many years, my own experience of gaining patients' permissions to use recordings of the music created during therapy sessions for teaching purposes has been surprising. Not once has anyone refused permission for recordings of their work to be used. On the contrary, most people are interested to hear feedback about what audiences thought and how they responded to what they heard, just as any musician might if recordings of their work were being used for the public to listen to.

The point to be made is that, in our experience of using the creative arts with patients at St Christopher's Hospice, we have been shown that both process and product can be equally valid. As part of our fortieth anniversary celebrations, we decided to set up exhibitions of patients' artwork in a variety of venues across the community within which we work. Patients and carers were both delighted and proud to show the work they had created publicly, and many of them were keen to view the work themselves and also to hear the comments made by others who viewed it. The exhibitions included work created in a variety of settings, for example creative group sessions, individual or family sessions in the home, art sessions held in care homes, health promotion projects with local schools and art created as part of arts therapy sessions. Even though none of our service users refused permission for their work to be shown – and if they had made known any concerns we would have been guided by them – the crucial matter is that it felt like a natural progression for everyone, having spent the time and energy creating the art, that it was then exhibited publicly.

Creating and planning an exhibition

Most palliative care services are linked to a specific geographical area, and within that area, there will be a number of organisations and venues which house art exhibitions. Most art galleries will be used to showing exhibitions of work by professional artists, but there is also a current drive for many of these places to extend and broaden their remit to exhibit work created by local community groups that will therefore be relevant and interesting to local people (Windsor 2007). We are now more likely to see periods of time devoted to displaying a range of 'community art' in galleries, created in education, health and social care organisations which exist within the galleries' local area. Planning for St Christopher's fortieth anniversary, we approached a number of venues within our local boroughs to request permission to exhibit patients' artwork. Such places included art galleries, libraries, civic centres and the administrative centre of the Mayor of London, City Hall. All of the venues that we approached were keen to work with us; however, we learned a great deal from the differing processes that we went through.

Important issues to raise when approaching a venue

- Agree the timing of the exhibition well in advance, as well as the dates and how long during the day and week it is able to be shown for.
- Agree who will put the exhibition up and take it down, what time the artwork will arrive and how you will gain access to the building.
- Ask about the area that will be available, the size of it and what kind of display material you will be able to use: things like exhibition stands, cabinets and picture-hanging materials.
- Ask if it is possible to use the opportunity to both raise funds for, and raise awareness of, the palliative care service.
- Ask if there will be any costs, if the venue charges for use of space, or if there are any issues regarding insurance of the artworks shown. A budget, sometimes only of £100 or £200, will be needed; its size will depend on a number of key facts such as whether there is a cost to using the venue, a cost in getting the artwork to and from the venue, a cost for hiring exhibition boards and materials.
- Make sure that what you agree is put down in writing, to avoid any misunderstanding.
- Identify a key person at the venue who will be responsible for overseeing the exhibition; keep in regular contact.

Selecting artwork to be included in the exhibition

There is no point looking for venues unless you have enough artwork to exhibit. Maybe the palliative care service will have accrued enough items over the years to collect them together and create an exhibition. We found that the relatives of many patients who had died were keen to loan us artworks for a period of time, so they could be included within the exhibitions. If some people did not want to part with the work of art created by a loved one, we made high-quality coloured copies of some paintings and used the copy in the exhibition rather than the original.

It could also be that a special arts project is set up in the palliative care service to create material for an exhibition. Sometimes patients can be motivated and energised if they know that the art being created is for a specific exhibition or there is a similar goal. For example, once, a group of patients in a hospice worked for over six months to create images on canvas. The theme was 'Stories of My Life', and over 40 paintings were created for an exhibition at a local gallery. There are many different possibilities when planning and arranging to exhibit artwork created by patients.

At St Christopher's, we are currently working on a project together with Dulwich Picture Gallery, a well-respected art gallery situated close by within our local community. The project, 'All our Lives – a Portrait of a Lifetime', has provided an opportunity for everyone associated with the hospice – patients, carers, staff, volunteers and visitors – to create their own portrait as a photograph. The project took place over a period of four weeks and will culminate in an exhibition of the photographs at the gallery. At the time of writing we are in the process of deciding how to exhibit the many photographs that have been taken and collected together over the weeks. One important discussion emerged when an artist involved in the project felt that only the 'best' photographs should be shown. Once again, we found ourselves drawn into uncomfortable territory where 'value', 'quality', 'talent' and 'aesthetics' were brought as issue. During these discussions, we realised that, for the hospice, we would never be comfortable for anyone or any photograph to be *excluded*, and that we would have to find a way for decisions about *selection* to be made. Of course, some photographs will technically be different from others, but we want the complete spectrum to be shown in the exhibition, otherwise only part of who we are and what we do will be shown. This is an essential priority at the heart of putting together such an exhibition: we must include all people's experiences of being part of the project in a way that shows each of the products as valid and worthwhile. The skill might be in the way that the photographs are displayed as opposed to the aesthetic quality of what is displayed.

A similar issue arises with other kinds of presentation. For example, Dives and Gill (Chapters 13 and 14) describe musical events in the hospice and local community. Do we employ only professional musicians? If so, we might be able to set standards of competence and styles of performance. If patients' or carers' performances are included our 'inclusion' priority might be relevant. For example, a hospice organised a professional conference at which patients who took part in a bell-ringing group performed alongside a staff choir. All the patients who were well enough and made the choice to take part contributed, but some who were physically and technically more able and felt safer to take a larger and more exposing part in the performance, and took part in a discussion that made the decisions. Musicians will be experienced in discussing with members of a performing group how able they feel to perform in public and choose material according to the level of ability.

Similarly, in our experience with participating in writing and performing drama, poetry or creative writing, it is possible for everyone to make a contribution, meeting our inclusion priority, while they may also be tactfully involved in the decision-making process.

Exhibiting patients' artwork

Displaying artwork within public venues is an art form in itself. For the exhibition to be successful, factors concerned with how the work is shown such as framing, hanging and positioning needs to be given careful thought and planning. Although the quality of experience people have when they witness an exhibition is always important, we must be able to identify what will be 'good enough' in terms of framing and displaying the art. It is not a good use of money to take patients' paintings to a high-quality framing agency which may charge between £50 and £100 to frame one painting, when a similar effect might be possible by buying frames and mounting board for between £5 and £10 at a local store. It is important to look around for the least expensive option that is appropriate to the purpose of the exhibition and the standing of the palliative care service when framing pictures, as the costs can soon mount up. An obviously cheap arrangement lacks respect for patients' achievements, while luxurious provision may raise questions about management of the service's budgets in an audience's mind. One or two volunteers working at the hospice might be experienced enough or have an interest in hanging paintings and arranging the exhibition at the venue. If so, they may be able to help the artist or artists with the physical task of putting the exhibition together. Hanging the exhibition and arranging the artwork at the exhibition venue can be hard and time-consuming work; it is important to identify who will be responsible for this. Also we must not forget that the exhibition will need to be taken down at some point. All of these things need to be thought about and planned in advance.

Celebrations and openings

Any public exhibition of artwork created by palliative care service patients will provide an opportunity for the organisation to be witnessed publicly. Inviting important guests to an opening reception or 'preview' might be a good way either to thank supporters of the organisation for past or ongoing contributions or to make positive contacts with the local community. It might also be an opportunity to invite representatives of local trusts to solicit financial support for future arts projects with patients or to invite the local press to report on the work that you are doing more broadly. As a result of an invitation to one of the St Christopher's fortieth anniversary community art exhibitions, a local trust committed itself to funding three community artists to continue their work with us over the next five years. This example highlights the importance of creating opportunities for patients' artwork to be witnessed, since, when the work is seen, it can sometimes generate dramatic and surprising responses.

Funding arts projects within palliative care services

Arts services within palliative care services are unlikely to be funded by statutory funding bodies in healthcare, notwithstanding the high value that a service might put on patients' creative work. Understanding why this is so and responding appropriately to attitudes in healthcare is important. We have suggested in other chapters that even if creative arts work is accepted as a valuable contribution, it can never be central to the healthcare objectives of palliative care service commissioners. Energy expounded fighting for statutory funding for such activities might be better used in other ways, such as identifying appropriate trusts, arts organisations and other private funding bodies whose aims and objectives might include supporting the use of the arts in such settings. This may mean tailoring applications so that they fit the priorities and assumptions of arts projects, rather than healthcare assumptions. For example, many non-healthcare arts projects employ part-time artists for a specified purpose and time, contracted for the project. Many artists are accustomed to having a portfolio of skills, activities and projects that they seek funding for, moving on to a new project as each is completed, or running several projects alongside each other. It is probably appropriate to the creativity and freshness of arts activities that funding aims at a specific project, product, exhibition or event. This contrasts with health and social care, where this pattern of project funding is often criticised for creating service instability because it does not contribute to long-term development of a service. So it is important to make a distinction between arts projects that are legitimately short term for good reason, and the funding of the core of arts provision in a palliative care service, which enables projects to be developed and sustained.

Funding applications to use the arts will differ in size, from supporting the salary of a full-time artist to backing a short four- or six-week arts project. However small or large the application, it is important to focus on a number of key areas. What follows is a simple guide to help put together a funding application for a small arts project, together with illustrations from an application that was successful with a small local trust.

1.   *At the beginning of the proposal, include a title. Make sure this is clear and concise. It is important to also include here who will be responsible for overseeing the project.*

Title: Creative arts groups for older people – a proposal to support older people within care homes through using the arts

Project lead: Day Services Manager

2.   *The second part of the proposal should include a concise background. This should provide some information on how the arts have been used as part of palliative care services in the past, or how the arts have successfully been used within hospices generally. References to successful evaluation and research that has been done are useful to support the effectiveness or value of the work.*

Background:

- Evidence and experience shows that people's relationship with the arts is heightened during illness (Windsor 2007).

- Over the past two years, using the arts has proved successful within the service and has enabled patients of all ages to have new experiences of themselves when they come to the end of their lives. These experiences have enabled people to gain a deeper understanding and clearer meaning of their own life, have provided a focus for the development of healthy relationships, and a means of enhancing and strengthening a sense of community.

- Due to a previous grant two years ago, we introduced the arts into the day centre. Through offering a range of creative arts groups, we were able to create a range of artwork which was recently exhibited to high acclaim at several prestigious art venues within our local community. As a result of these exhibitions, we have been approached by a number of organisations caring for older people within our local community to see if we would be able to offer some creative arts sessions for their residents.

3.   *The next section could include some information of how the money you are requesting will help the hospice to build on what it has learned from its past successes.*

Building on success:

- The hospice has developed and implemented a range of creative arts possibilities for patients and their carers as part of the day centre. During the past two years, due to the success of our existing arts project, our artist has also managed to work with a number of patients on our inpatient ward. Many of these patients, during the final days of their lives, have created art products which have been given to their loved ones as a keepsake.

- We plan to build on our successful programme offered within the hospice building.

- This additional funding would allow us to bring the arts to people who would not otherwise have access to such a life-enriching experience within the places where they are living and dying.

- There is evidence to point to the increasing isolation of elderly people, due to geographical distance from family, or from limited family or other social support, and to a lack of provision of specialist palliative care to these people in the last weeks of their lives.

4. *It is now important to give a brief outline of how the project will be structured – explaining the length of the project, how the sessions will be offered and plans for sustainability when the funding comes to an end.*

Structuring the project:

- This project will take place over a 12-month period.

- We will extend the creative arts opportunities available to patients within the hospice to a neglected group of people coming to the end of their lives.

- Creative arts sessions will be delivered within the care home environment in order to support residents' psychological and social needs and to enable a deeper expression of meaning, identity and community.

- We plan to offer an introductory package of sessions to a group of care homes across the community that we serve. This would include two creative group sessions for residents, and an introductory creative group for care home staff. Our aim would be for the care homes to experience the benefit of such creative arts sessions for their residents and to examine further the possibilities of the continued funding of sessions from the care homes themselves.

- We plan to audit the project in order to identify how many care homes take up the possibility of buying further sessions for themselves and also to prove the efficacy of such work. We also plan to offer our findings to similar organisations in order to provide a template for future work.

5.   *The final part of this simple funding proposal should include a breakdown of the budget. As well as including a breakdown of payment costs for the artist involved, it is important not to forget the costs of arts materials and, as the work is to take place within the local community, the costs of travel.*

Budget:

- Cost per group session   ****
- Material costs   ****
- Travel costs   ****
- **Total**   ****

6.   *If it is possible, include copies of artwork created in the past, as the majority of the time the reality of witnessing the work will be more important than the application itself.*

Using the arts as part of promotional material

Although exhibiting patients' artwork within community settings will promote the work of the hospice, there are many other ways that art produced by patients might be used to enhance the image of the organisation.

Including images of patients' artwork, having first secured their permission, within the service's annual report or other publicity material can be an important way to motivate and inspire the general public to get involved. With the growth and development of the worldwide web, patients' artwork can also be shown as part of the service's website. Again, this will take the work produced to a wider audience. Also, with the progress and improvement in the development of digital equipment (see Chapter 8 on digital arts), we are increasingly presented with new and easier ways to capture and demonstrate the value of both the patient's work and the arts projects that we undertake. The production of a simple DVD can be a useful way of putting together a brief report of how an arts project has been developed and completed. Such a product can be used to accompany future funding proposals so that grant-making trusts can witness what is possible, as well as staff using the DVD for teaching and educational purposes.

In whatever way they are used, images of patients' artwork can be an important tool in raising awareness and raising the profile of the palliative care service, as well as creating interest and inspiring positive responses to the use of the arts themselves. Exactly the same points might be made about participation in events such as open days, bazaars, celebrations and dinners, where performances representing art, music, creative writing and drama can all make a contribution. Similarly, it is important to look out for opportunities of participation in community events. For example, for some years St Christopher's has participated with a local music festival, providing a small-scale venue for an afternoon concert. This connects the hospice with a local organisation and potential local supporters, helps musicians to feel that they are making a contribution to an important local service when they give their performance, and provides an event for day care and inpatients to participate in. Connected with these, it makes the hospice feel like a normal place and may help potential patients, carers or relatives feel comfortable with the hospice as a place of care for family members in the future.

Working in partnership

The possibilities of exhibiting patient's artwork within local venues, or developing opportunities to work together with other organisations that are part of the community that the palliative care service serves, provide chances to work together in partnership.

Over the last five to ten years, a number of arts organisations have been set up in order to offer palliative care services the potential of using artists to work with their patients. The MAP foundation (Petrone 1997) is a very successful example of such an organisation. It is the inspiration of Michele Angelo Petrone, who was an artist and cancer patient. He had the vision of offering creative arts workshops to patients coming to the end of their lives and also to their formal and informal carers. The work produced as part of these workshops is then exhibited to raise awareness of the work and what can be achieved.

Although there can be great benefits from joint ventures, such as gaining experience of new possibilities for what a palliative care service might offer to its users, and working together in partnerships will be increasingly important for palliative care over the coming years, it is important to raise some fundamental questions before embarking on any agreement with arts organisations:

- As we have seen from the experiences mentioned already in this chapter, the artistic product can be an important asset for the palliative care service. It is important to understand how the artistic products created will be used in the future. Will the organisation you are working in partnership with expect to use the artwork as part of their promotional material? This will be important as you both might want to use the material to raise funds and awareness in the future and you might find yourselves competing within the same arena.

- Most arts organisation will only fund work for a short period of time. If your organisation is expected to take over the funding of a project in the future, will the partnership organisation still require you to use their name? Again, if you are applying for funding for this to happen, you might find yourself in direct competition with the partnership organisation.

- When entering into partnership with arts organisations, it will be important to be clear about the management structure within the initial agreement. You will have a knowledge of what is or is not possible within your own community in a way that the partner organisation will not. Therefore, it will be important that you are able to manage and guide the process of the work at all times.

Working in partnership with such organisations can be rewarding and extremely beneficial in providing arts experiences for patients and introducing new services into palliative care. However, such partnerships do not come without their problems and it must not be seen as a cheap option. It is vital that palliative care service management teams provide a clear and transparent strategy for the future direction of the organisation. Every palliative care organisation and the communities that they serve will have their own unique possibilities for developing and providing the future end-of-life care that is needed. Entering into a partnership with an arts organisation must both serve and underpin these possibilities, otherwise the hospice might just find itself benefiting the partnership agency, whilst gaining little in return.

Conclusion

This chapter began by asking some questions about the place and meaning of the arts within society. As healthcare institutions are part of that society, the same questions must exist when we introduce the arts into them and use the creative arts with those who operate in other social arenas. The comprehension of the value of both process and product in terms of the arts is crucial when we come to understand and identify the value of creating art with people who are ill.

Whether the artist is working as a professional within their own studio or is coming to the end of their life with a terminal illness in a palliative care setting, the act of creating can be a powerful, motivational occupation (Hartley 2007). Also, the product created can be as astonishing as it is rewarding. Whoever the artist is, it is important to understand, acknowledge and give the opportunity for the creator's need for it to be shared, witnessed and valued.

Further reading

Ansdell, G. and Hartley, N. (2000) 'The legacy of music therapy', The programme of the Annual Conference of the Association of Professional Music Therapists and the British Society for Music Therapy, February.

Bunting, C. (2007) *Public Value and the Arts in England.* London: Arts Council England.

Hartley, N. (2007) 'Resilience and Creativity.' In B. Monroe and D. Oliviere (eds) *Resilience in Palliative Care.* Oxford: Oxford University Press.

Petrone, M.A. (1997) *The Emotional Cancer Journey.* Brighton: ESBH Health Authority.

Windsor, J. (2007) *Your Health and the Arts.* London: Arts Council England.

Websites

www.artscouncil.org.uk – website of Arts Council England, highlighting their work, procedures and criteria for funding application and publications, accessed on 13 February 2008.

www.mapfoundation.org – highlights the work and publications of the MAP Foundation, accessed on 13 February 2008.

www.apmt.org – website of the Association of Professional Music Therapists, accessed on 13 February 2008.

www.bsmt.org – website of the British Society of Music Therapy, accessed on 13 February 2008.

www.baat.org – website of the British Association of Art Therapists, accessed on 13 February 2008.

5 Research and Audit in Palliative Care Creative Arts

Malcolm Payne

Evaluating creative arts in a healthcare setting

You look at a painting, view a video, feel a sculpture, listen to music. The product of a creative arts process is valued by the experience of its audience or viewer. You work with clay, paints or a camera, with a pen or a group of actors. The process of creation is valued by the experience of its producers. There are well-established critical norms for how to analyse artistic creations, which can be applied to work done in palliative care settings. Why do we need to think in a different way about creative arts in palliative care?

There are two reasons. One is that although a high standard may be achieved by patients working in creative arts, they are not professional artists, neither are they students in arts education. Therefore, their work needs to be assessed by an appropriate standard relevant to the aims for engaging them in creative work. If it is about reminiscence, their work's nature and power will need to be different than if the aim is artistic self-fulfilment, therapeutic engagement or another objective. Moreover, a palliative care patient is affected by serious symptoms of advanced illness; their work must be evaluated with consideration for the emotional and physical limitations of their condition.

The second reason is that a healthcare setting, such as a hospital, hospice or day centre, is established to provide health and social treatment and care for people with health problems. It is not a studio for the creation of artistic achievements or products. Therefore, evaluating the role of creative arts in palliative care, or as part of any healthcare service, raises questions about what we are examining. Moreover, creative arts are a new incursion into palliative care and healthcare practice; even the various arts therapies are fairly new in their impact. The chapters in Part II show that artists daily face uncertainty and doubt from their colleagues about what they do and whether it is worthwhile. Looking at the *Journal of Medical Humanities* suggests that the main focus of work in the humanities, literature, art and drama especially have been on how the humanities reflect medicine and healthcare experiences. A perspective on the contribution of the arts to treatment is largely absent. Yet there is an established literature on bibliotherapy (self-treatment and psychotherapy using reading of literature; Bolton and Hedges 2005) and art, drama and music therapy are well-established techniques, even if they are not commonly available in the UK National Health Service.

How, then, are the contributions made by creative arts to palliative care and healthcare to be evaluated? Should it be on the same basis as other healthcare interventions are evaluated, such as their efficacy in relieving medical symptoms? One of the important ideologies of palliative care practice is holism, the principle that people's treatment should respond to all their needs as human beings rather than focusing on a limited range of symptoms. Therefore, their need to express creativity and to use creative arts to achieve self-fulfilment and other social and psychological objectives is relevant to what palliative care aims to do, as well as healthcare needs.

This chapter argues that to help in establishing the role and contribution of creative arts in palliative care, and in healthcare more generally, research, audit and evaluation work needs to concern itself with demonstrating the value of creative arts interventions and helping to select appropriate interventions for the particular circumstances and needs of palliative care patients. At the same time, we must consider how to incorporate into healthcare evaluation and research the particular aims and methods of creative arts work.

Research, audit and evaluation

Research, audit and evaluation are connected. The overlap is that they are all concerned with investigation; the differences are about the aims of the activity. It is important to think through precisely what you are trying to achieve in carrying out a study, since you may be demanding more of yourself than you need to for your objectives. Carrying out research properly is a time-consuming and precise activity, whereas all you may need is an audit or evaluation that can be a bit more 'quick and dirty'. Thinking about what your investigation aims to do is the first step towards sensible advance planning.

Audit is about good planning and management of your service; evaluation is about proving yourself and your work overall; research is about developing knowledge and understanding about your activity, in this case, the creative arts in palliative care. To put it more precisely: research is a systematic and rigorous process of inquiry that is disseminated so that it contributes to human knowledge and understanding. Audit is the planned process of collecting and examining information about services to decide whether stated criteria are being met. Evaluation is the process of examining a service to decide whether it is achieving worthwhile objectives. The major difference is that research is about creating new knowledge, while audit and evaluation are about understanding what is going on now; that understanding might be new knowledge, but that is not necessary for it to be useful in running or seeking funding for the service. Research is disseminated and preferably published, while audit and evaluation are more often used to inform management or funding decisions. Audit aims to check that what should be happening is happening and what should not be happening is not, while evaluation is concerned with seeing whether what is happening is worthwhile, bearing in mind the wider aims of the service.

Audits may be continuing or focused. Continuing audits involve collecting and reporting information regularly, while focused audits concentrate on a particular aspect of service. Statistics are collected regularly to enable palliative care services to report on their work to interested parties, usually commissioners of services such as primary care trusts, local authorities or charitable foundations. This is also a report back to ourselves, it summarises the achievements of our work for a period, allows us to look back with satisfaction or to think how we might do it better next time. The St Christopher's practice is to ask each department of the hospice to identify part of their work each year for a focused audit. Seeing such a requirement, you might try to avoid being chosen, since it might involve a lot of work but, equally, you could clamour for inclusion because it might offer the chance to make a case for your work more effectively.

An example of setting up a new palliative care arts service demonstrates the difference in practice. Audit would involve planning the regular collection of statistics about patients served and the feedback they give about the benefits and problems of the service. A focused audit might enable a part of the service to show how much work it is doing or how successful its outcomes are. Evaluation would collect this information after a period and look at how the service has developed to see if it met the aims set out in the application for funding or contributes to the service's strategy. Research might be mounted to examine the process of interaction between the artists and patients, or look at the effect of artistic work on the patients' interaction with their families.

If you are setting up a new service, or developing a new element of service, it saves time, effort and heartache to be clear what kind of investigation you need to provide evidence for funders and your colleagues about the value of what you are doing or to plan your work effectively.

Research governance in health and social care

Research governance is the way in which research in an organisation is managed so that it contributes to the aims of the organisation, is carried out ethically and is efficient in meeting appropriate objectives. For example, a palliative care service would be unlikely to agree to research that involved stressful questioning of sick inpatients because, however useful the information it provides might be, this would be contrary to the overall purpose of the organisation in helping people to die in comfort. It also treats patients unethically and probably would not achieve the objectives set. The English Department of Health has a policy on research governance in health and social care; documents about this are available on a specialised website (see the list of websites at the end of this chapter).

The requirements include:

- a mechanism, which includes wide consultation, for deciding whether a research project should be undertaken in the organisation, setting any funding and requirements for the project and managing the interface between the organisation and the project
- a process for managing research projects that are established
- a mechanism for managing the reporting and disseminating of outcomes, so that when we have done the investigation we can do something about what we have found.

The process at St Christopher's Hospice is fairly typical, and I describe it here as an example. Staff or outside researchers that want to carry out a research project draft a proposal setting out the research aims and questions it seeks to answer. The research committee considers and approves this, or advises on suitable changes. The committee includes clinical members of the senior management team, people interested in research and, if they are not otherwise included, a representative of the main clinical departments. It also has an external academic representative.

Usually approval is subject to the researcher receiving research ethics committee approval from the relevant NHS committee. This is a complicated process; a long form has to be prepared and submitted to the committee. Guidance and the relevant forms may be found on the website of the National Research Ethics Service (NRES) of the National Patient Safety Agency (NPSA), whose addresses are listed at the end of this chapter. Its staff and the people who chair the local committees are helpful sources of advice.

If you have negotiated these approval processes, at St Christopher's the proposal goes to the hospice research and audit committee, which is an open meeting of staff, attended mainly by middle managers, such as ward and home care area managers. They look at the practicalities of achieving a research project. For example, they will decide on the best way of recruiting patients to be investigated, and give advice on the content of questionnaires. At the same time, a senior management team member is appointed to liaise with outside researchers to help them gain access to the information and contacts they need in the organisation.

When the research is finished, researchers give a presentation at the research and audit committee, so that people who helped to organise it or helped find respondents can get feedback on what the research found. It is a condition of approval of a project that results are published, if at all possible, and the research committee helps less experienced staff doing research to prepare publications for journals, professional magazines and conferences. Senior staff also look at proposed publications in draft, to check information given about the hospice is correct. The hospice library collects publications that result from research done at the hospice.

Methodology and methods

Your methodology is the strategy by which you want to explore your topic. The main choice is between what are sometimes called quantitative and qualitative methods, although this is in some ways a false dichotomy, because you will almost certainly want to include both. Hidden behind the quantitative/qualitative distinction is a debate about epistemology, that is, how we know whether something is true or not. Broadly, there are three views of truth and knowledge.

Some truths come from the authority of tradition and experience. In many situations, we look to established ways of doing things and experienced people to identify what works best. Much professional practice is expressed in advice, guidelines, policies and procedures based on accumulated experience of what colleagues or managers have found works in a particular situation. This is the only way of applying understanding of the limitations of a building or an organisational system to more general knowledge. Such guidance often comes from politicians or managers implementing a decision about their aims in the best way possible. The previous section on research governance is very much like that: it points to official guidelines and procedures, and gives an example of how a particular system works that has been found to be effective in one organisation. The sources of tradition have often been important sources of authority in society: the state, the church or the law.

Other truths come from rigorous observation of the world to see what consistently happens in defined situations. This has led to the development of 'scientific method' and is sometimes called positivist or realist, because it assumes that there is a reality that can be observed and understood independently of it, by a neutral observer. The aim is to describe and then explain why and how that reality happens. So, when they are painting, how do artists represent the colours that they see? We would need to have ways of measuring the colour seen and the colour represented; there would of course be many shades and depths of colour. We could specify these in various ways, using Pantone shades, for example, but in a very complex picture this might be difficult and we would also have to specify the overall effect in a patch of paint achieved by the combinations of various colours. We would need to look at the artist's techniques, selecting and mixing colours. We would also need to understand how colour is perceived and processed by the eye and brain, and how brush strokes represent the texture of the real world. Many of these things can be measured, but we would also need to understand variations; for example, the work of a number of artists are thought to indicate that their perceptions were affected by eye disease (Emery 1997). From this brief example, you can see that to be a neutral observer in this way means being very rigorous in taking every possible factor into account. To produce a complete account of the real world, you have to find ways of measuring very complex data. Even then, there will be human variability, so some of the time we will be saying, using statistics, that there is a range of variation and that in this circumstance one thing is more likely, while in another the outcome is likely to be different. Using these techniques of rigorous observation, we want to make statements about how the real world works that will hold true for all relevant situations. In particular, we want to explain the causes of things in detail, so that we can make sure we understand why things work as they do. Biomedical research tries to use this approach to getting information, because when we are dealing with human life and death, it is important to be sure that the treatments we are using are effective. If drugs or surgery do not work, then we might cause damage to people. Hence, biomedical professions place great emphasis on research of this kind.

The third kind of truth is called 'interpretivist' and refers to a lot of information about human beings and social life; it is particularly important in the social sciences. The perspective says that all information is processed or 'interpreted' by human beings, and how they process it is partly 'constructed' by their social experience, their culture, their expectations and their values. There never can be a 'reality' in many areas of knowledge, because human psychology and society intrudes. Social construction asks: 'Why did you choose to ask this (research) question? Did it come from assumptions about the world that are true only for your culture or your particular moment in history or people of your particular upbringing?' Interpretivists prefer to use research methods that are reflexive, that is, they recognise that the interpretations of many different points of view are all 'true' to that person or social group, and research should help you to understand all the different points of view, instead of your expecting to come up with one view that is 'correct' or 'true'. This sort of approach often means that you can get a more in-depth or complex picture of what is happening.

These different views of truth would lead you to different ways of doing your research. However, there is a political issue here. Positivists and interpretivists are doubtful about each other's methods. Positivists expect concrete results about well-specified issues that tell you whether something is true or not, while interpretivists think that the process of being rigorous and specific means that human complexities and differences are hidden or avoided. Positivist methods are necessary in biomedical fields to allow us to be clear what is effective and safe in achieving results in surgical techniques and medication, and this means that people in biomedical fields tend to assume that this kind of knowledge should apply to everything. However, I would argue that interpretivist methods are much more appropriate to creative arts work. This is because doing creative work means interpreting the world, producing an outcome whose impact is again interpreted by its audience. The process of doing it and viewing it is an important aspect of the value of the work, which we have to set alongside any other possible outcomes. People working on creative arts in healthcare need to argue for this position to inform the research that they undertake.

However, we have to accept that being part of healthcare services means that we have to identify what healthcare outcomes our work may achieve and produce evidence that what we do achieves them. Otherwise, why should anyone pay for them? One answer to this might be that in every aspect of life we should expect to have opportunities for creative achievement; some would say it is a natural part of life. While this might apply to healthcare, as elsewhere, it might well be argued that healthcare services should not pay for everyday creative opportunities. Therefore, we have to show how creative opportunities enhance healthcare.

Any appropriate research methodology for creative arts in palliative care, therefore, needs to build an approach that looks both at measures of artistic achievement and of healthcare impact. Creative arts research is likely to be interpretivist, concerned with the process of creation and interpretation and psychological and social responses to it. Healthcare measures are likely to be more positivist, concerned with evidence of improvements in response to other healthcare interventions: feeling better, slowing psychological and physical deterioration. It is important to identify the value of creative arts in an overall experience of life for patients, their carers and people in general. Outcomes from audits, evaluations and research may be able to show that there is a valuation contribution to the achievement of the holistic philosophy of palliative care, even though specific health-related benefits are hard to prove.

Accepting this, we can look at the various methods available from research textbooks, such as the two recommended in the further reading at the end of this chapter. These fall into a number of types (adapted from Robson 2002):

- *Document analysis* – identifying trends, issues and information contained in existing documents; if we looked at hospice annual reports, for example, we could find out how many mention creative arts work and the role it plays as part of their work.

- *Observation* – watching activities going on and identifying outcomes that we can see; if we watched a number of different arts groups, we could describe people's behaviours and reactions and possibly their skill development.

- *Surveys* – asking people through interviews or questionnaires about their experiences; for example, we could ask people about their attitudes to their arts work, how they value it compared with other treatments they receive, which activities they prefer, and any impacts that they can identify on their lives. We could also ask people around them, for example other professionals or family members.

- *Tests and scales* – this special form of survey allows us to compare reactions from our respondents to the typical responses from other people to a standard set of questions. For example, the Hospital Anxiety and Depression Scale (HADS) is a well-known scale for testing how much anxiety and depression people in healthcare situations experience.

When the initial collection of data has been achieved through these and other methods, we can analyse the information; again there are many techniques that we can obtain from research texts, but the outcomes will be:

- *Descriptive* – information that will allow you to describe the work and its outcomes that you do more fully or in a better way. For example, you may be able to say how many of different kinds of patient you serve, and what they and their families feel about their arts work.

- *Analytic* – information that will enable you to analyse the work in ways that explain how or why something is happening. For example, you may be able to say why colleagues are referring or not referring patients to you, or whether there is any improvement in psychological reaction to advanced illness among your patients, compared with people who do not receive arts service.

- *Identification of further issues and actions* – nearly all research tells you that you need to know more, and leads you to the next project to fill the gap in your knowledge, but it may also guide you in some professional action. For example, you may have found that male patients prefer one kind of approach and female patients prefer another. This presents you with other choices. You could restrict what you offer to the people who prefer it, or you could try to get males, females or both to change to accept both approaches.

Deciding on methodology and methods presents you in theory with many choices, but the limitations of your type of work and the people you serve may determine what you can do. If you are doing something fairly concrete, you may be able to do an analytical study that shows how much better your patients do than those who have not had your service. If what you do is more nuanced or complex, you may be able to show a variety of reactions and analyse them better than you could before doing the study.

Building research credibility

A number of aspects of a project will enable you to build credibility for a piece of research or evaluation. One of these is selecting a mix of methodologies and methods appropriate to what you are doing. There is little point in trying a complex statistical analysis of patient outcomes, if your arts service only aims to make a contribution to part of the psychosocial services in a hospice. This is because other factors will affect patients' outcomes, many of which may be more important than your contribution. You may, however, be able to demonstrate improved happiness and a sense of achievement among patients, and positive attitudes to being able to have creative experiences. A number of aspects of any research project are likely to be able to build its credibility to have a impact on others.

Advance planning

Research and evaluation need to be carefully planned in advance to cover all the aspects of the service that you want information about. Useful elements of advance planning are as follows:

- You should identify research aims and research questions. It is useful if research aims are expressed in a way that makes it clear when you will have achieved what you are setting out to find out. For example, I have sometimes seen a research aim that starts: 'to explore…' a topic. However, most topics have infinite implications, so it is always difficult to decide when you have completed a task like this. It is better to start off with words such as 'identify', 'explain', 'understand' or 'evaluate', because if you set out the topic clearly, you clarify and set a limit to what you are going to do.

- Research questions are different from aims; they try to express precisely what you want to find out. The most useful way of thinking about this is to try to express what you don't know clearly. For example, I did a literature review (now published as Payne 2006) to 'identify' (the aim) the social objectives that writers about palliative day care said it should achieve. My research question was: 'Do professional articles about palliative day care distinguish social objectives for the activities in palliative day centres from other kinds of objectives?' (Answer: yes or no, and I gained some information about what social aims they considered.) The reason for doing this was that researchers had suggested that social rather than healthcare aims were more relevant to saying what the aims of palliative day care was, but social aims had never really been researched.

- Based on the research aims and questions, and a literature review (telling you what is already known) about the topic, you can then work out your methodology (your strategy for researching the topic) and what methods you might use (how you collect the information).

- Then you can write a proposal to explain what you intend to do to explain it to the organisation you want to do the work in (see research governance which explains that you will need such a document to gain approval to carry out your project).

Independent involvement

One of the important ways of building credibility in any research is to think about the balance between independence and reflexivity that is appropriate for the topic. To show clearly that the service and its outcomes are the result of your achievements and not the topics you have chosen to research and the way you have chosen to research them, it is important for the people involved to be independent of what they are researching. You can achieve this by consulting widely about the design of your project, so that there are a variety of different views about your methods. The person asking the questions, distributing the questionnaire or analysing the results may also be clearly separate from the person providing the service. This means that respondents can make adverse comments without feeling that they might hurt your feelings when you've worked so hard; on the other hand, if they feel bad about you, they will not perhaps feel so strongly that they need to get back at you, so you will get a more balanced response. Finally, when you are reporting back, or writing your publication or report, you can get a 'peer review' – that is, people like you who know about this kind of work look at it to check if they can suggest ways of improving it, or look for holes in what you have done.

While independence is important, reflexivity may also be crucial. You cannot get at many truths by having neutral outsiders do the asking, because patients and carers in their troubled lives will expect researchers to convey a sense of engagement and commitment to their needs. It is perfectly appropriate to gather personal views from written information or from people involved, but this will be more credible if it is collected consistently and in a planned way. For example, if you are going to collect your own observations from an art group, you improve credibility by carefully defining what you are going to collect and having a format that allows you to collect it in a planned and consistent way. Similarly, if you are going to interview people in a fairly open-ended way, you need to have a consistent system for analysing the themes that they talk about. This allows people to understand the impact of your involvement on the data that you are collecting, and allows you to collect data that you might not have noticed in the ordinary way but which are revealed by having a consistent pattern of information. On the same theme, if you are going to describe your own experience then recording it consistently will help to show patterns up; you can see an example of a personal journal in Chapter 10, which could be analysed consistently to produce themes. You could get even more information if you asked the whole arts team to keep such journals and analysed them consistently.

Counting

People involved in arts activities may reject counting as a way of evaluating their work. It is not necessary to get into the complexities of statistical analysis, for which you need specialist advice; it is important to set up the research in advance to make it possible. However, counting is possible in the following ways:

- Count the number of people served or involved in an arts activity, or the number of people attending a group event or exhibition. This is a measure of support giving credibility by showing how much support there is.

- Ask people to rate activities or their attitudes, feelings or responses on a scale of one to five or one to seven. This enables you to put a figure on slippery aspects of responses to complex aspects of your work.

- Count the number of times something happened. For example, if you are using an arts activity to help people express their feelings, count how many times people talked about their emotions or certain words were used. If you are trying to help people learn skills, or promote their engagement in the work, count how many times they used the skill, or note the length of time they worked on their pot as compared with the amount of time they gossiped. This sort of counting can demonstrate or confirm commitment, interest and outcomes.

- Compare what happened in one situation or with one population and what happened with comparable people. For example, did an arts project have the same effect on both men and women, or were the patients receiving creative arts help less anxious or depressed than similar patients who did not experience it? Doing this requires careful planning of the statistical work needed to make valid comparisons, and of the number of people that you need to test. This means at least getting statistical advice or asking an experienced researcher to plan the project for you.

Writing up

How you write up the project will have important consequences for its impact. An internal report can only affect colleagues, but it may be important in gaining support for your work. Publication more widely requires deciding on an appropriate journal, or rewriting it for several. For example, you would choose a palliative care journal to have an effect on palliative care colleagues or an arts journal to influence colleagues in that field. You might choose a professional journal if you wanted to influence practitioner colleagues, or a more academic journal to add to the knowledge base that will eventually affect decisions about the political acceptability of arts work in palliative care.

Literature reviews and searches

Literature reviews are an account of information you gained from a literature search, that is, an examination of the existing writing about a topic that you are interested in. The principle of doing this is that any development of knowledge builds on what has been found out before; otherwise it just repeats existing knowledge. It is also a waste of time doing research to find out something that is already known.

There are three reasons for doing a literature search:

- to find out useful written information about an unfamiliar topic; this also helps you to see different points of view and later on will enable you to teach or write a publication or report and recommend useful and worthwhile publications to help other people's learning

- as the basis for a research project, because any research needs to build on what we already know

- as a research project in itself to bring together comprehensive information about a topic.

Literature reviews start from what you already know. You probably receive journals and own books on professional topics. To build on these, you can visit an academic, professional or public library. Ask the librarian how to find things that you want. They are trained to do this and usually welcome an interesting inquiry, but they will leave you to do your own searching, because you have to take responsibility for it.

Starting from the most recent and comprehensive book or journal that you can find, list all the references on topics that are of interest to you, and then go looking for these. Do the same with these, and carry on until you cannot find references to anything that you have not already seen.

It is wise when doing this to keep a careful record in your notes of the reference of the publication. If you want to refer to it later, you will need to find it again, and if you want to refer to it in a publication about your research eventually, you will have to 'cite' it; that means inform people how to find the article to get more information, just as you have done in your literature search. You will have to do this in a standard way, that each publication sets, so it is crucial to save yourself time later to keep detailed notes to enable you to produce this citation in the correct form. This means a note of the authors, the date of publication, the title, the title of the journal or book an article appeared in, the volume and number of the issue of a journal, or the editors, place of publication and publisher of a book and the page numbers of the article in the journal or book.

The problem with doing a literature search by following back from a known publication is that you may get stuck in a single track. I recently read a piece of writing by a nurse looking at transition of seriously ill children into adulthood, across the division between children's and adults' services. She had assiduously found all the very sparse healthcare literature about this topic. However, she did not realise that careers guidance professionals interpret their work as transition from school to work, and there is a huge literature, with concepts and research about that transition that would have helped her. Therefore, you should try a little serendipity. If you look at the library list of topics, pick some general subjects related to yours and check through the shelves on those topics to see if you can find anything of interest. For example, if you are a music therapist, you may be used to looking at the music shelves and psychotherapy. You could try looking at education or social work to find material in related topics. Just wandering through the library and looking at unexpected shelves or journals you do not usually view may bring a new insight to you. For example, the same music therapist may not usually look at the economics shelves, but there will be some work on the economics of the music industries.

Computer databases automate the searching process. Two kinds exist:

- search engines, which give you access to information on the internet

- specialised databases produced by academic institutions and libraries covering a specialist literature.

Search engines such as 'Google' are familiar, although for doing research you may find the specialist engine for academic work, Google Scholar, more useful than the general engine. It is important to evaluate the quality of the information, since anyone can put things on the internet. Edited journals have quality control because someone has evaluated the usefulness and relevance of the contribution to a particular topic. This is true of academic and professional journals if they are peer-reviewed (two or three people who know something about the topic have looked at the publication and agreed that it is worthwhile).

The specialist databases do, however, present problems. First, you have to identify the topic accurately in one or two words, because the computer indexes rely on 'keywords'. I once did some research on 'missing people', for example. I asked someone who had written a book about it and he said there was very little literature, so I was not surprised when I came across few articles and books, most of which I already knew. However, one of these mentioned the term 'runaways'. When I searched for this word, I found hundreds of articles, including some on runaway nuclear reactions, which gave me a conceptual sidelight on running away.

A second problem with computer searching is that it is mainly useful for articles. This is, again, because indexing relies on keywords or 'abstracts', the summaries written by the authors of articles. Longer pieces of writing are less fully summarised, and chapters of books are sometimes not included in indexes. For similar reasons, the most comprehensive indexes are about fairly concrete scientific topics. Although most libraries have OPACs (Online Public Access Catalogues), which cover their whole collection and allow you to look for books, there is very little detail. You can search most university library catalogues for books; a good choice is a university that you know has a course in the subject you are interested in. Also you can search on the internet the catalogues of major public libraries like the British Library (www.bl.uk) or the (American) Library of Congress (www.catalog.loc.gov).

Case study: music therapy as an example of a creative arts audit

In Chapter 14, Gill provides an example of a comprehensive audit in creative arts in palliative care, and we can use this example as a case study to consider the factors that will have impact on any similar exercise. To examine this audit critically, we have to look at the following:

- An analysis of the source of the impulsion to carry out an audit, since this will tell us something about the political situation in which the work was carried out and into which the report of the audit will make its way. Chapter 14 describes an audit where using music therapy as an intervention in palliative care was new, there was an externally funded project where the money would run out, and there was an existing commitment to carry out an audit to demonstrate the value of music therapy and justify seeking further funding.

- The methods the audit used, in order to give its report credibility in that political situation. Gill made sure she worked through research governance approval processes carefully and that there was an independent element in all the evaluations that she arranged. However, she does not shy away from using personal feedback and experience as part of the study, appropriately for an arts evaluation.

- The outcomes achieved, and their impact on practice and decisions. Gill carefully sets out positive responses and achievements from a variety of points of view. This might have more credibility if it was more analytical and critical, looking for points of criticism and ways of improving what was achieved. The account would also be strengthened if the therapist had an organised scheme of observation. It may be useful to devise a recording system to note observations consistently.

Conclusion

Research, evaluation and audit are crucial parts of creative arts work in palliative care for two main reasons. One is that creative arts work is a relatively new aspect of service and needs to justify its position. The second is that its way of thinking about the world is different from the predominantly biomedical approach of the healthcare services within which palliative care is positioned. The research approaches in palliative care are dominated by a biomedical positivist approach, because of the particular knowledge needs of this professional world. People doing research and audit in the creative arts needs to acknowledge the reality of that scenario and organise their research to contribute to the need for creative arts work in palliative care to justify itself within the way in which the palliative care world looks at evidence of achievement. However, in doing so it is important not to deny the nature of creative arts work and its aims. The arts are concerned with interpretation and therefore research methods appropriate to creative arts work in palliative care need to acclaim and incorporate the value of more reflexive research methods.

Further reading

Addington-Hall, J., Bruera, E., Higginson, I.J. and Payne, S. (eds) (2007) *Research Methods in Palliative Care.* Oxford: Oxford University Press.

An edited book, but the group of editors are leading contributors to palliative care research and contribute many of the chapters. An authoritative account of methods accepted within palliative care, showing how they might be applied in palliative care work.

Ansdell, G. and Pavlicevic, M. (2001) *Beginning Research in the Arts Therapies: A Practical Guide.* London: Jessica Kingsley Publishers.

A widely used book on research in an important creative therapies.

Hart, C. (1998) *Doing a Literature Review: Releasing the Social Science Research Imagination.* London: Sage.

Hart, C. (2001) *Doing a Literature Search: A Comprehensive Guide for the Social Sciences.* London: Sage.

Two excellent books on carrying out a literature review and literature search.

Robson, C. (2002) *Real World Research* (2nd edn). Oxford: Blackwell.

There are many texts and practical guides on how to do research, but this is a particularly comprehensive and well-regarded one, useful because it focuses on researching situations in the real world, rather than constructed research, such as experiments.

Websites

www.dh.gov.uk/en/Policyandguidance/Researchanddevelopment/A-Z/Researchgovernance/index.htm, accessed on 15 February 2008. The English Department of Health research governance website, which includes the latest research governance framework for health and social care, guidance and notes about good practice.

www.nres.npsa.nhs.uk, accessed on 15 February 2008 – The website of the National Research Ethics Service website of the National Patient Safety Agency, which manages the research ethics approval process.

Part II

Experiences of Creative Arts in Palliative Care

6 Experiences of Creative Arts in Palliative Care – Introduction to Part II

Malcolm Payne

Part II contains a series of chapters written by members of the arts team at St Christopher's Hospice, describing and analysing their work, to illustrate and extend the account given in Part I of creative arts work in palliative care. By including contributions from several members of the same team we aim to give a picture of the potential of a broad arts service to achieve interactions and cross-fertilisation between different approaches and elements of the service. We do not seek to present a 'St Christopher's approach', but to show instead a variety of possibilities at different levels of complexity, seeking to achieve a range of aims in different settings.

Some principles demonstrated

This book proposes that a principle of creative arts provision in palliative care is that it should respond to the needs of the patient and their family. The creative arts is not about self-fulfilment for the patient or self-indulgence for the artist; it is designed to contribute to an overall healthcare service for patients and their families. It should also contribute to the community's experience of help in and engagement with death, dying and bereavement. Therefore, what patients and their families need should set the criteria for the arts selected and how they are used.

One of the important variables is the setting in which creative arts are provided. This has often been in day centres. However, we have argued in part I that helpful provision is possible in a range of settings. The chapters present work in several different settings: a day unit, at the bedside in a hospice in-patient unit, in patients' own homes, and in care homes. The practice described is transferable between many of these settings. For example, Dobbs (Chapter 10) describes visiting the bedside in the in-patient unit with an 'art trolley', and Hearth (Chapter 11) describes taking a choice of art materials to patients in the community. Dives and Gill (Chapters 13 and 14) offer a variety of musical instruments in a music room or by taking them to people's homes. These examples of practice illustrate the practicality of offering choice of media in which to work, which may be achieved in any setting. As Hearth (Chapter 11) points out, the bedside is a setting in people's homes, in care homes and in in-patient units.

Behind this practicality, another important principle, explicitly stated in several chapters, is the importance of choice of media if patients are to reach their creative best. Even where the subject is a starting-out point, like Harmer's elephants (Chapter 7), interacting with the media is a crucial way of building creativity, while for the arts and music therapists (Chapters 10, 13 and 14) interacting about the media enables communication between therapist and patient.

The chapters also demonstrate the principle that the skills and creativity of the artists are crucial aspects of success. The contributions therefore all start out by explaining something of the authors' attitudes to creative arts in palliative care, what they see creative arts contributing to this setting, which guides them in their practice. In the case of Butchers (Chapter 8), this is to reject a self-identity as an artist, and claim the identity of craftsman. In other chapters the writer explains something of what creative arts mean to them in their lives, as a foundation for their practice. Moreover, from practice with patients emerges awareness of and commitment to the place of art (and craft) in their own lives. We see how their own creative work contributes to freshness and renewal in their work with patients.

Similarly, most of the chapters also show the importance of participation in a team of people with commitment to providing a creative arts service and effective professional supervision, and how this helps them to make their contribution while maintaining their own personal motivation and mental health. The example of Hearth's personal journal (Chapter 11) demonstrates how she manages some of the personal and interpersonal consequences of this work for herself and the people around her, both at work and in her personal life. Such a device may also be an important basis for critical reflection on practice and therefore of professional development

The work sometimes has a pattern; for example, Harmer (Chapter 7) and Butchers (Chapter 8) describe working with groups of patients or individuals moving from well-established starting points, and Tasker (Chapter 9) has a consistent pattern in the way she builds up shared projects. Both arts and music therapists use an introductory meeting to build a picture of patients' starting points and preferences, and to build confidence in their capacity to make a beginning. Moreover, many authors stress the importance of selecting activities to achieve early success to provide motivation for uncertain patients and families. In addition to that, the arts therapists select activities that they think will fit the personality and needs for therapeutic expression of their patients.

A comprehensive creative arts service in palliative care

The chapters in Part II distinguish between different aspects of a comprehensive creative arts service in palliative care. There are at least four elements, as follows:

- Part of the service offers an opportunity for creative expression and occupation as part of involvement in a palliative care setting. This may simply contribute to the programme of a day- or in-patient setting to occupy patients and family members with a stimulating, fulfilling and worthwhile activity. It may avoid boredom and give them interesting activities to talk about at the time and later. Another purpose may be to divert patients' and family members' minds from daily concerns about their illness or social problems. It may also be the beginning point in further adventures in creativity. Sometimes working on creative activities may offer a setting in which people may learn social skills in interacting with others. For example, people might see how others talk about dying, or present their illness in conversation, and this might help them in talking to family, friends or neighbours about difficult topics. The activity might be an opportunity to get into a conversation in which they can test out their own feelings and responses to their illness or the effects on their family. Sometimes it may be possible to share experience directly, for example to discuss with another patient or family member how they talked to young children in the family about the fact that they are going to die.

This aspect of the service begins Part II, since it is most comprehensively described in Chapters 7 and 8 by Harmer and Butchers. They discuss how they motivate and engage diffident patients, select tasks that permit easy beginning of achievement, and lay the foundation for future development. These approaches are perhaps the most replicable in less comprehensive creative arts programmes.

- Involvement in an individual or group activity to achieve an artistic product has the aim of patients or family members using time to gain personal self-fulfilment. Because patients in palliative care have limited time left to them in their lives, and an important principle in palliative care is 'to live until the moment that you die', doing something worthwhile in that time is important. Yet the illness often means that patients have little energy to pursue more active interests, if they have enjoyed sport or keeping fit or travel, for example. They are usually unable to work or do household chores and pursue their normal leisure interests as they used to do. Many creative arts can be managed with the smaller stores of energy that patients have and, as these chapters show, they can achieve good results even with limited skill in the early stages of their artistic development.

Chapters 7 and 8 demonstrate aspects of this element of a creative arts service, particularly in how patients are helped to take on bigger projects or work together on a joint project. However, this aspect of the service is most fully expressed in Tasker's discussion of her work in digital arts (Chapter 9) and in the development of the shared projects she describes. Of particular note here is how different arts and skills can be integrated into one project. Although the photography project primarily uses a flexible visual medium, for example, it also stimulates intellectual and language development through writing poetry. Similarly, the experience of the fashion show also stimulates written expression in poetry. In this way different media are enabled to have their different impacts, as various audiences may respond differently.

- Individual or group psychotherapy is a more specialised provision needed by fewer patients. This process uses the creation of an art object, and the process of achieving it, to engage the patient or family member in interactions with the therapist. These aim to resolve psychological and emotional difficulties that are preventing the patient or family member from dealing with other social issues in their lives.

The practice of arts therapies in palliative care are explored most fully in Chapters 10, 13 and 14. The authors examine the issues presented in palliative care by the short timescale during which the patient can develop work, and the tiredness and other symptoms that may limit what they can achieve. While the emotions and social concerns that their predicament presents them with may also be a limitation, involvement in creative arts may provide them with an opportunity to deal with personal and family issues in a new and unexpected way.

- The fourth element is the community arts, discussed directly by Hearth, Sands and Dives (Chapter 11–13), but also by Gill (Chapter 14). These chapters show how individual work with patients can interact with broader community artistic activities in the palliative care service and local community.

In presenting these four elements of an overall service we do not suggest that every palliative care service or health and social care agency will want to offer all four. Each of these elements can be provided separately to contribute to par-ticular health and social care objectives. However, these chapters all illustrate another important principle of this book: the importance of development and progression as part of a creative arts service, whatever it offers. Unless patients are helped to make progress in what they can achieve artistically, and the projects and activities that they take part in therefore progress, change and renew themselves, the creative arts will not contribute to therapeutic benefit, but will be a mere time-filler.

Responses and feedback

Each of the chapters also comments on the responses and motivations of the participants. A consistent theme is how past life experiences, particularly in education, have made people feel that they are no good at art; that they cannot achieve worthwhile results. It is disappointing that arts education a generation or two ago had this effect on people's capacity to engage in artistic activity as part of their lives. One of the social gains of pursing creative work in palliative care is that it may contribute to a wider recognition of the value of artistic endeavour for everyone among members of the public who see the work in exhibitions. Family members, friends and neighbours may experience through the patient how valuable artistic and creative work may be in responding to social and psychological issues in our lives, and be more prepared to acknowledge its value and take it up themselves in the future. In this way, direct work with patients may indirectly enhance family and community resilience. The chapters show how the authors address the issue of patients having been turned off art, and get patients working, achieving results that are better than they expected. This is a necessary skill if a creative arts service is to engage with patients, do worthwhile rather than routine work, and if it is to help them progress in skill and achievement.

These chapters also illustrate in various ways the importance of seeking and receiving feedback from patients and the public about their experience of the creative arts process. For the arts therapists this is integral to the therapeutic process in which they are engaged. For all the artists, but particularly those working in group settings, it allows them to gauge and manage the development of the group's work. Feedback from audiences, the public and professional colleagues is an important marker of the achievement of an arts programme, and, listened to carefully, allows us to identify particular aspects of an activity that were more or perhaps less successful to an audience or to participants. Formally organised feedback through audit and research also allows the people working in a creative arts service to report back to its funders and its colleagues and gain support and critical engagement in what it is trying to achieve.

7 Pottery and Painting

Lynn Harmer

Pottery, art and palliative care

I was 15 when I first discovered clay. I made a model of my dog and instantly fell in love with clay's soft and receptive nature. Following school, I trained as an art teacher and extended my experience of clay through a postgraduate diploma in ceramics at Goldsmiths College London. I have had two pottery studios, one in Devon and one in Peckham, South London, producing domestic ware and containers for plants. Although my early teaching experience was at primary level, I was asked to teach pottery in an adult education setting where I still work today. My involvement with students with learning difficulties or disabilities (SLDD) grew over a number of years, and as a tutor with a local community college I have worked in a number of healthcare settings and with a wide range of client groups. I came to palliative care by chance when a friend working in the NHS persuaded me to apply for the post of arts facilitator. I have now been working in palliative care for nearly ten years and together with the patients have enjoyed a number of fulfilling projects, two of which I will describe in detail.

Starting off

When our hospice patients first arrive to join a group they may feel nervous or apprehensive but they are nearly always curious and open to what others have achieved. The work they see around them speaks for itself and they see how creative other people, who are in the same situation, have been.

After they have had a look around, I usually suggest we begin with something simple. A common first reaction is for patients to say: 'Oh, I won't be able to do that', so I have developed projects that break the activity into easy-to-follow steps. I always start with a demonstration of each stage and work with them, supporting, encouraging and affirming their first attempts. Their initial apprehension is rarely a block, and as they see the object emerge, their enjoyment and confidence grows. After they have achieved some results, they turn to others and say: 'It is amazing what you can do, you don't know until you try and I have been really surprised about what I have been able to make.'

Creating an elephant

We have found that a good starting point in pottery is creating an elephant. This particular project works well because the models don't have to be perfect to be seen as a good result, in fact they seem to have much more character if they are irregular with one leg a bit shorter perhaps or a lopsided ear. It is not perceived as an activity that you have to get absolutely right. The examples the patients see beforehand of other patients' work are all very different. Elephants may look old, young, playful or sad and as the elephant emerges so does its personality. Above all, there is the interaction with whoever else is involved. In a group there is comparison, joking, story-telling and laughter. It may also become an occasion to share painful or troubled feelings as the elephant becomes the vehicle for communication. Elephants seem to symbolise many different things to people but in particular the notion that 'elephants never forget' becomes potent at the end of life.

I demonstrate the activity using specific pottery techniques such as pinching and coiling rather than sculpting or modelling. Pinching means gently squeezing clay between finger and thumb and coiling means rolling clay using fingers to stretch and form a long even coil of clay. Often, I introduce it by saying that I am going to show them some simple techniques, which will ultimately be useful in making other things, thus suggesting a creative future for them. We work hand-in-hand throughout the whole process together. I demonstrate Stage 1 and we do that together and then move on in incremental steps. An elephant probably takes someone a single session of 90 minutes.

The method

We start by forming two golf-ball size pieces of clay from which we pinch two separate thumb pots, one of which is slightly larger at the rim than the other. The two bowls are joined to form a hollow egg by pulling the clay of the larger bowl over the rim of the smaller one. It may look like a knobbly potato rather than a smooth egg but this can add to the character. We make it hollow because it dries more quickly and uses less clay, and is therefore less likely to blow up in the kiln. For the same reason you have to pierce this hollow egg of clay with a small hole, so that the air is not trapped. We usually do this right at the end in what has become the under belly of the creature.

Stage 2 is making the elephant head and trunk together, as it is much stronger this way. The process is one of gentle squeezing and pinching, so the clay trunk grows out of the head. The head may start by looking like a dinosaur and gradually turns into a duck shape. As the creator feels their way and becomes more sensitive to the pressure needed, the trunk gradually grows and can be twisted up or down. There is a saying that if you want to welcome good fortune you have the trunk curled upwards and face your elephant to a door or window.

We make the legs by gently squeezing another golf ball of clay into a sausage, and then gently rolling it with the fingertips on the table, so that it becomes even in thickness. The height of the legs will depend upon the size of the elephant. The legs should be fairly thick and all the same height so that the elephant will stand steady.

Joining all the pieces has to be done well. It is vital to create a texture on both parts that are going to be joined so that the clay bonds like glue. More agile patients can use a potter's knife and scratch both surfaces before adding a little water with a toothbrush. Patients with less dexterity may use just the toothbrush to create mud on both surfaces. The head and legs are put into place, mud onto mud, so that they stick to the body.

As they are the most fragile, the ears are the last things to go on. Patients choose at this point whether to have an Indian or African elephant and, interestingly, most people choose the latter, which has larger ears. Usually, when you put the ears on, the elephant really does come to life. We take two marble sized pieces of clay about the same size. Then holding on to one edge, flatten it and make it as thin as you can. It needs to be floppy, like thin elephant skin. To attach the ears, we blend the bit we have been holding onto when we made the ear into the side of the head, so that the ear goes back against the side of the head.

Finally we create the eyes. We look at the elephant full on, and using a thin pointed wooden stick (kebab stick or end of pen is fine) we position them either side of the trunk, trying to get them equally balanced. If we feel the elephant needs a mouth, we insert a wooden tool under the trunk to create the bottom lip. Last of all, we roll a little bit of clay in the hand to make a thin worm and put the tail on. We used to make tusks but they can be fragile and break off in the drying. If tusks are desired, it is possible to make two holes and then glue in bits of plastic curtain hooks after the elephant has been fired.

Firing

I ask patients to put their initials on the base of the elephant's feet and explain that I am going to let it dry naturally. The superficial moisture dries off in two days and the elephant is fired slowly in the kiln for a further two days. It will probably be about a week before owners see their elephants again. When they do, the elephants will be changed into resilient pottery.

The patients are given the option of adding on some form of decoration usually in the form of a glaze; this makes it endure longer, making it stronger and more waterproof. I use brush-on glazes since patients can apply the decoration as though it were paint. Mostly, we use earthenware glazes as they are easier to apply and fire. Sometimes after the glaze firing we adorn the elephants with jewellery or tapestry silks depending upon the character of the elephant that has emerged.

Leaf dishes

Another achievable project and one that will take no more than an hour is making a leaf dish. Patients choose a leaf from the garden; we make suggestions because we know which leaves will produce the best pattern.

The clay is rolled out on a cloth to stop it sticking to the table. We use wooden guides on either side of the clay on which the rolling pin must roll across to ensure the clay is an even thickness. This prevents warpage and splitting in the drying and firing stages. Patients are then asked to lay the underneath of the leaf into the clay. Most clays are a very receptive medium that can pick up the finest detail, which is often far more subtle, accurate and appealing than if drawn by hand. We check that the imprint has taken by lifting the leaf at one corner and then cutting around the shape of the leaf. As cutting to the leaf edge can destroy the detail and look messy I suggest leaving a one-centimetre border around the leaf which can be pinched thin with finger and thumb to imitate leaf structure. The clay leaf is then laid into a plaster or fired clay mould that is the right size, incline and shape for that particular leaf or for its particular function. As the leaf still is on the clay, you can gently push the whole object down into the mould without leaving fingerprints. Then we gently remove the leaf and admire the results. The stem can be pulled over to form a handle.

After the first firing the patients would choose a glaze which both protects and enhances their dish. The choice partly depends on whether they intend to use it with food or as decorative piece. There are glazes advisable for either purpose.

Developing pottery

A whole range of developments is possible from these simpler techniques. Sometimes the group is happy to work on a project together. At other times, patients prefer to work on individual projects of their own design and inspiration. One patient took easily to the technique of coiling and developed the theme of re-creating coiled pots from past civilisations. He researched various cultures and made many splendid coil pots using a wide range of shapes and decoration.

Other people choose to throw on a potter's wheel. We have had people who have shown great promise and tenacity, although patients later in their illness maybe less able to engage in certain techniques that are physically demanding. Most wheels require the thrower to 'saddle' the seat although there are a growing number of table-top and 'user-friendly' wheels that are more comfortable. The technique does require the maker to lean their body weight over the wheel and coordinate hands and feet in different activities as you would when driving a car. It is possible to work together and for the facilitator to take responsibility for part of the process such as operating the wheel or providing one of the hands. It is possible to have the pleasing sensation of 'centring' with a very small piece of clay that can represent feeling at one and in control of something at a time when things may feel very chaotic.

Starting painting

I help beginners to approach painting by teaching a technique called 'wet on wet'. The first step is to cover the paper with clean water and then apply the pre-mixed wet paint to the wet paper. The advantage is that you get striking effects straight away, which can be very encouraging. People usually come to the painting class from one of two camps. Some have had a positive experience of themselves as a painter or can draw well. Others may have had negative experiences at school or have never had a go. However, most patients who come to the group seem to be curious and consequently are open to the experience, especially when they have seen other patients' work adorn the corridors.

The method

The majority of people don't feel confident about drawing, so I try to eliminate any need for that from the start. We begin with a composition, usually a simple seascape based on a painting I have done myself as a sample. In the first session, we cover some pointers: foreground, mid-ground and distance with far-away things being cooler and paler, and nearer things being darker and more in focus; we discuss spaces such as two-thirds sky and one-third sea.

We use good quality watercolour paint and paper so that colours are vibrant and the paper doesn't distort. I always suggest painting the sky first so patients cover two-thirds of the paper with clean water. Then, with the paint already mixed, we would apply the colour. We mix the main colours in the palette but often find the colours also blend into each other on the paper and create fabulous effects.

When this section has dried, we use the technique of 'wet on to dry' paper. Quickly dragging a small amount of paint across dry textured paper leaves some of the paper clear and white, which appears as sparkling light on water.

The final stage is to place a few details to help us 'read' the picture. This might be a suggestion of coastline or usually a boat moored in the bay. Often there will be a couple of gulls in the distance. These are completed in a tone of grey that silhouettes and positions them nearer or further away helping us to feel a sense of distance and perspective.

In this process, patients are able to achieve a pleasing result very quickly and easily and feel more confident to move onto other challenges.

Developing painting

We have had people who have been professional artists or have pursued art as a lifelong hobby. One patient, for example, had done a lot of pencil drawing in his life but was wary of painting, so it was very interesting for him to work without drawing at all. The benefits were that this was quite freeing for him and he has developed an impressive 'Turneresque' style with very little pencil preparation. He now feels he has many more options for his creative spirit to explore.

Although some people prefer working from still or real life, beginners often prefer to develop through copying from other artists' work, photographs or the samples I have created showing step-by-step progression. The samples take people through a sequence of techniques and levels of difficulty and give examples of how to interpret visually the world around them. Patients are learning through example and when ready will often bring in a photograph they wish to interpret themselves. This is broken down into light and dark perspective and colour. We discuss why the patient chose this photograph and what they most want to capture in their own interpretation. The trick is to keep it all as simple as possible. My input in this process is based on my observation of both the artistic and psychological performance of individuals. Occasionally, I witness frustration and performance anxiety as patients start to feel as though they are not achieving what they want. In these situations we re-examine other techniques that are more achievable. We read each situation on its own merits and always return to what has already worked for the patient.

Motivation, recognition and responses

I have noticed a difference in attitude between the patients who choose to do pottery and those who gravitate to painting. The 'would-be' potters are more curious and less likely to have set expectations about what is going to happen or how successful they will be. It is possibly that many people have not experienced pottery at school and are therefore not prejudging their performance so are able to be more open. There is the element of 'I feel like a kid again' and they are more willing to 'play'.

In marked contrast, the potential painters have usually had a positive experience of painting or drawing and are willing to build on that. Those that have been told they 'are no good at art' won't even consider painting. There is an argument here for providing a range of mixed media and presenting patients with an opportunity to do things they have never done before.

Even so, I have observed that the majority of people will try most things at least once. Finding themselves in an uncertain time in their life can bring about either a need for more control and safety or an attitude of 'What have I got to lose?' The team has discussed the role of uncertainty in our work. If we, as a team, can work with uncertainty, we may be role models for our patients, who are living with uncertainty and there would be greater capacity to explore death and therefore make the most of life that we have left.

I do not attempt to measure what is going on. I listen to what people say about how creative activities have opened up their experience of themselves and how their family and friends see them changing and feed back to them; a sort of ripple effect. Kennett, Harmer and Tasker (2004, p.254) wrote:

> It is possible for a patient to experience him or herself in a different way – not only as a very sick person but through this new and different activity as a person who can have influence on materials and the surroundings and make something pleasurable and lovely.

Through the creative work, patients seem to have a fuller experience of things around them. Recently a patient told me that since she has started painting landscapes, she now notices the sky and its changing mood and colour. She said it was 'like having new eyes'.

Some patients' families are hungry for the creations they bring home. Many patients arrive with commissions for more saying: 'My daughter did not believe that I had made it and now my other daughter wants one.' Another patient said: 'Goodness me, I am this person who can create things and could even be called an artist.' Patients are proud and flattered when we ask if we can borrow their work to put on show in the hospice or in a wider exhibition elsewhere and relatives even prouder when they visit and see the displays. It's as if the family see their relative in a new way, a positive discovery that can enhance the relationship and family dynamic. I witness people whose self-worth is growing and who are challenging limiting self-definitions around illness and dying.

I am aware that some projects might be gender-biased and appeal more to some than others, so it is important to ensure there is choice. People's artistic priorities express their personality and interests. For example, one patient only wanted to model horses' heads; throughout his life he had enjoyed both working and looking after horses and had tremendous respect for them. His work was serious and accurate in all details and his passion influenced other males in the group, one of whom took up a similar challenge.

A recent change to the way we work is having the craft and painting groups working in the same room at the same time. Originally the crafts were elsewhere and the two groups were very distinct. When the groups merged the craft group were concerned that they would be expected to paint and were a little guarded. The painters also were concerned that they would lose the quiet meditation and contemplation of their practice. Undoubtedly the atmosphere is different and there are implications for how such a group is facilitated but interestingly there has been unexpected migration of 'craft' people who have seen what the painters are doing and have said: 'Oh, can I have a little go at that?' I observe people who are convinced they can't paint, gain confidence through copying and creating the designs they achieve in the craft. They also see fellow patients new to painting producing pleasing results on their first session and this encourages them to have a go. One female patient who had worked with crafts for a long period made the transition into the world of painting and amazed herself with the results she seemed to produce almost unconsciously. It was a different experience for her and she and her family were constantly surprised and delighted with the paintings that emerged. Following her demise, her family members were so attached to her paintings that they drew lots to make sure the work was distributed fairly.

Another patient who had achieved a high standard in his work was discharged and together we found alternative art classes he could attend. When his illness returned and he came back to the hospice art group, he reported that he had not learnt as much in the other group, because he felt safer here to make mistakes or to take risks, rather than having to make progress with formal techniques.

One of the reasons for this kind of reaction is that the groups provide a safe and supportive environment where staff and patients offer cooperation and camaraderie. It feels as if everyone enjoys each other's creative journey and there is a very strong feeling that we are all sharing the same experience. Even though they might be doing different work, patients take an active interest in the endeavour of other people and what they are going through. Patients have an experience of themselves as being alive and creative who are learning and producing something new and vital instead of being someone who is ill and less useful in the world.

Projects and groupwork

I like to design new activities, because it keeps me fresh and this is passed on to the patients. I like to introduce one or two new projects every year, although for individual work, leaf dishes and elephants remain the most popular. Sometimes I suggest the group works together on one piece. The groups seem to quickly form a cohesive identity even though individuals may come and go, and it is rare that I have known a group not to get on. Groups have been very responsive to contributing to the hospice environment and enjoy the camaraderie of a joint approach. We have had a number of pottery projects, where the whole group works together over a period of several weeks. In one case, we magnified a diagram of a seed head. This was broken down into a series of interconnected shapes which patients constructed, glazed and fired before reassembling and fixing onto a felt background. This presently adorns one of the walls in the main reception area.

Group projects can take many forms but common elements include individual creations that contribute to a bigger picture. One of the first projects attempted in the pottery group was a tile plaque designed to adorn the outside wall where patients arrive by ambulance. Patients opted to create a 9" × 3" × 6" tile plaque using the hospice movement symbol of sunflowers. Patients 'played' with different ways of producing sunflowers using a wide range of pottery techniques eventually opting for an appliqué approach where clay is added to hand cut tiles. Every participant made a tile either of a sunflower or adjoining stems and leaves which collectively joined together to make an emblem of life and colour welcoming new patients on their arrival.

Case study

The case study used here to illustrate the positive nature of this work is one in which I was personally involved and has been previously cited in an article by Kennett *et al.* (2004).

The patient, a middle-aged man called Michael, had been admitted to the inpatient unit suffering from acute back pain. This particular symptom was proving difficult to control and I was asked to visit him to discuss his interest in painting. This was not an unusual referral and I have worked with a number of patients who are experiencing acute symptoms of pain or anxiety. Although Michael had not painted since he was at school, it was something he had always meant to take up, and we subsequently spent an absorbing time mixing paints, experimenting with colour and trying different painting techniques. During this period, he seemed to be largely unaware of his back pain and he was eager to plan other times to work together. The nursing staff observed the reduction in the severity of Michael's symptoms during these sessions and asked if there was any way we could involve Michael's ten-year-old son Joe in these occasions too.

For a wide variety of reasons, Joe was finding it difficult to visit his father at the hospice and both the staff and Michael's wife were concerned that Joe and his father might not have any quality time together before Michael's death. Joe had a passion for all art activities and with a promise of joining in an arts project, he was persuaded to visit the hospice after school. On arrival, I gave Joe the choice of which activity he would like to work on with his father and without hesitation he chose to make a baby elephant out of clay and persuaded his father to make one too. The session that followed was a delight to experience. They followed the step-by-step approach described above and both laughed and teased each other as their lumps of clay changed from dinosaurs to ducks and finally into elephants. The final creatures were given much praise and mutual admiration and congratulations passed between father and son. When I took the elephants away to the kiln room Michael was showing Joe his paintings and, glancing in later, I observed them quietly painting together. After a sudden and rapid deterioration Michael died a few days later. Although I didn't meet Joe again I was able to pass on two sturdy baby elephants for Joe to keep: lasting symbols of shared moments with his father.

Kennett *et al.* (2004, p.256) report:

> Feedback about such sessions include patient enjoyment, lifting of mood, calming anxiety, relief of boredom, pride, achievement and pleasure at being able to make a gift for a relative or friend. Patients have been appreciative of the individual attention they have received and conversed with them freely whilst working. Sometimes they have talked about their love of the arts and at others have shared some of the things that are worrying them.

Equipment and resources

The clay we use needs to be responsive and tolerant as it is used in a wide range of projects by a wide range of people. Some clays can be temperamental and may splinter and break. The buff stoneware clay we use has been tried and tested over many years and has proved itself to be extremely reliable and resilient.

We use earthenware glazes as they have a lower melting point and therefore fire at a lower temperature. This means that firings are cheaper and faster and we can provide a quicker return of work to patients and their families. Earthenware glazes, although may they lack the matt subtlety of the stoneware glazes, are easier to apply, melting more evenly to give pleasing results. The firings are carried out in a top-loading electric kiln that can fire and cool in two days.

The painting class supplies good quality watercolour paper ($300g/m^2$) and artist-quality watercolour paints to make sure the paper does not buckle and the colour does not fade. A wide range of brushes are available that offer some of the properties of expensive sable at half the price. Many companies offer cheaper alternatives and we have found the artificial fibre may be longer-lasting.

8 Craft Work

Adrian Butchers

Craft and art

I have always been involved with craft work as a personal interest, but I don't see myself as an artist. I think there is quite a difference between doing craft and being an artist. I have had a go at watercolour painting, which is not my strong point. Craft is more controlled than painting, and it is perhaps easier to gain confidence in doing it. For many years, I ran my own business in various service industries. I work in the Creative Living Centre, and the hospice has paid for me to go on a number of courses to build up my knowledge and skill. There are many courses in every locality. I worked making wedding cakes for about 30 years, and I occasionally teach the patients sugar craft.

Starting points

The most popular crafts with patients are mosaics, painting on silk and painting on glass and porcelain. We do card-making and sugar craft occasionally, where it connects with patients' interests or the time of the year. I try to keep developing new activities or joint projects and finding new designs that patients can try; it keeps me fresh if I am trying something new regularly.

People will come to the craft group in the day unit without having much experience or knowledge, but mosaic and silk painting allows them to start right away and achieve a successful product within a morning. Therefore, these activities are very suitable for a general activity group in a day unit. We also find them easy to take to the bedside or to people's homes, for patients who are unable to come to the unit, as the craft can be placed on a tray on the bedside table. Then if they are involved with the activities over a period, they may move on to more complex work. However, many patients are happy to repeat products that have been successful for them; for example they might make silk scarves for several family members.

Attitudes

My approach, which is to see myself as a practical craftsman with an interest in a range of activities, often strengthens the confidence of patients to 'have a go'. Many people do not know what to expect, and are quite nervous. They have been made to feel that they cannot do something like this at some time in the past, often at school. Some patients actually say: 'When I was at school I was rubbish at art, I was rubbish at craft, so I am obviously no good.' Part of our aim is to enable them to feel that they can achieve something, to feel fulfilled. When they actually make something, the look on their face is wonderful to see. The sense of achievement that they have is inspiring. They are very proud when they take it home.

We always make it clear when they arrive at the group for the first time, that nobody is forced to do anything. If they can just sit and observe, then we can gently bring them in if they want to. In the craft group, they are very supportive of each other. A lot of the patients will encourage new patients without our intervention, they will say: 'When I first came I couldn't do anything, but now I'm doing this.' They will always encourage others to have a go.

There is no gender difference in patients' preferences in craftwork. There have been two or three men who I judged wrongly, thinking that they would not want to get involved in art and craft. We had one recently who said: 'No, it's not for me.' He made no secret of the fact when he came to look at the craft, that he did not think it was for a man. However, after watching other people get involved he eventually said: 'I think I could.' Because we made him feel that it was all right just to observe, he became more confident to the point where he wanted to join in. He started off with a mosaic mirror and then he said he would really like to do a mosaic coffee table. He has produced an amazing coffee table in mosaics, amazing because of the complex design and the care he took to produce a good product. He took home a template on paper of the size of the table and designed the pattern himself. It involved him using a compass and the intricate design consisted of overlapping and curves. He transferred the design using carbon paper to the tabletop. He chose the range of tiles and colours he wanted very carefully because he wanted it to be used in a particular room in the house. He took a lot of care in making the mosaic and worked on it for a few weeks, and he was justifiably very proud of the finished piece. His wife was astonished at his achievement particularly as he had never attempted any craft work before in his life.

Mosaic work

The two easiest options to start off with, if somebody has not done mosaic before, is making a mosaic picture frame or mosaic mirror, because they do not involve cutting any of the tiles (see Box 7.1). We buy the basic picture frame and patients can use the tiles whole to edge the frame. They will achieve this in perhaps half or three quarters of an hour.

Box 7.1 Mosaic work

Mosaic mirrors
Materials

> Mirror
>
> Pre-cut medium density fibreboard (MDF) board
>
> PVA glue
>
> Small paint brush
>
> 20mm × 20mm mosaic tiles
>
> Grout
>
> Small spreader or spatula
>
> Sponge

Process

We have the MDF board pre-cut to 13" × 13" (your local DIY store will do this for you) and use small square mirrors from IKEA as you can place three rows of tiles all around the mirror in the pattern of your choice without any of them having to be cut. First fix the mirror to the centre of the board with PVA and allow to dry. The tiles can then be placed in to position and stuck with the PVA glue. We have found the best method is to attach the tiles around the edge of the board, making sure they do not overlap the edge of the board and then continue working towards the mirror. Allow at least 24 hours for the glue to dry before grouting. The powder grout is mixed with water to a thick creamy consistency making sure there are no lumps. This is then spread over the tiles making sure all the tiles are covered and the gaps filled. When the whole area is covered, scrape off the excess grout and with a clean, damp sponge wipe over the front of the tiles gently. Keep rinsing out the sponge. It is important all the excess water is squeezed out of the sponge. When the mosaic is clean, leave to dry. You will find it will have a dusty appearance. This is easily removed with a soft duster. Screw two eye hooks in to the back of the board, attach picture, wire or cord and the mirror is ready to hang.

Mosaic picture frames
Materials

> Narrow, flat, pine picture frames available from IKEA in an assortment of sizes. The range is called RAM
>
> 24mm × 24mm unglazed ceramic tiles available by mail order from Mosaic Workshop. These come on a sheet of paper of approx 200 tiles and are easily soaked off

PVA glue

Small paint brush

Tile grout available in a range of colours from Mosaic Workshop

Small spreader or spatula

Rubber gloves

Process

These tiles fit the width of the frame exactly so no tile-cutting is required. If you are using more than one colour of tile for your frame it is advisable to place them around the frame first to ensure you have the effect you want. It is important that you leave a small space in between each tile to allow for grouting. When you have decided on the design, stick them on to the frame using PVA ensuring they are level with the edges of the frame. Allow the glue to dry thoroughly before grouting the piece, as with mirrors.

Mosaic coffee table

Materials

Flat pack coffee table from IKEA. We use Fornboro which is 45cm diameter and under £7.00

Mosaic tiles

PVA glue

Small paint brush

Grout

Small spreader or spatula

Tile nippers

Goggles

Paper and pencil to draw out design

Carbon paper to transfer design on to the table

Compass (useful in designing the pattern but not essential)

Process

The process is the same as for the mosaic mirrors. Transfer the design to the table top using the carbon paper. Some tiles will have to be cut using the tile nippers. Always take care when doing this particularly with glass tiles; it is advisable to use goggles. When all the tiles have been stuck, allow to dry for 24 hours. Then follow grouting instructions as for the mosaic mirror. Attach the legs.

We carry a good range of colours and two types of tiles: ceramic, which offers much softer colours with a matt finish, and glass, which have bright vibrant colours. Glass offers the whole spectrum of colours; the glass ones are brighter because the tiles are shiny. If we could only fund one type of tile, I would go for glass rather than ceramics: there is a larger range of colours and they are more vibrant, which the patients seem to prefer. The wide choice makes it interesting seeing what somebody will choose; this can be a useful start in conversation. Two ladies in my present group enjoy working on mosaics and always pick the reds, oranges and greens; other people will go to the ceramics and choose the beiges and browns, the softer colours.

We stick the tiles with PVA onto just very basic flat plain picture frames in one of two sizes. The width of the picture frame is exactly the same size as a ceramic tile, so there is no cutting involved at all. Therefore, when we take it to the bedside we don't need tile nippers or other equipment; the tiles can be stuck straight on to the frame. When the adhesive is dry, we put a layer of grout over the top to fill in the gaps. It comes in a range of colours that patients can choose between. If patients are able to do it, they will do it themselves.

Case study: Jack

Jack, a man with motor neurone disease, had very limited mobility. When he first came I did not think he would engage in any art and craftwork because he worked in a very senior trade union post in a public service; I was proved wrong. By setting him up with a lap tray, he could just move the tiles to stick them on. His first mosaic work was a picture frame. Unfortunately, while he was here, his 11-year-old grandson died. Jack then launched into making picture frames for every member of the family to hold the picture of his grandson. He came once a week and every week, when he was brought in, he knew exactly what he wanted to achieve that day: another two picture frames for family or friends to put the grandson's picture in, eventually completing over a dozen frames. He did advance from that: the last project he worked on was a coffee table that he wanted to do for his wife in Newcastle United colours. We managed to get the Newcastle logo to put in the middle of it. His wife had no idea that he was making this for her and he just managed to finish it. He was picked up by volunteer transport, took it home and gave it to her; she rang the day unit to thank us. It was his idea; he wanted this for her, having worked through all the picture frames for the family.

Painting silk scarves

Another good starting point, which interests many women patients, is painting silk scarves, because they can achieve a finished article in half to three quarters of an hour and take it home with them on the first day. However, men also become very involved and will make one, take it home, give it to their wives and then come back the following week with a list: 'My sister wants this colour.'

The process is to start off with a basic white silk scarf (see Box 7.2 for details). We will give patients a colour chart that has a range of 36 colours and recommend that they use three or four. You can start confidently without any particular artistic skill, because you just drip the colour on with pipettes, a little dropper that has the dye in it. The dye does all the work for you; the colours run into each other. You put the scarf onto the table, spray it with water and then just gently pleat it up so that it is not completely flat.

We use a range of steam-fixed dyes; you generate steam to fix the colour. In most cases, we use a rice steamer and a microwave to generate the steam which fixes the dye and makes it colourfast. You can also do it in a colander over a saucepan of boiling water. You can use iron-fix dyes, but then you have to wait for the whole scarf to dry with the dye in it before you can iron it. It does not produce the same effect and is not as instant as with a steam fix; at the beginning or for occasional craftwork, steam fixing allows patients to see instant results from their work.

As a development, you can also create patterns. When the dye is on and still wet you can sprinkle table or rock salt onto the scarf. This draws some of the dye back out again into the granules, forming feathery patterns in the dye.

Developing silk painting

If, through doing the starting projects, people build up an interest in silk painting, we go on to painting pictures in silk (see Box 7.2). As a craft, silk painting is much easier than it looks. Many patients are reluctant to use paper and paints but find they are able to express themselves with the freedom of the flowing gutta lines used to draw on the silk. Painting the silk is easy as the colours flow naturally and wonderful effects and colours achieved. If the patient is still unsure of drawing they can always paint an abstract or geometric pattern – even very simple designs look good on silk. There is no need to worry about getting it wrong as a mistake can very easily be changed into a success by drawing another gutta line and painting over the colours.

A suitable project is to produce silk painting that can be mounted and framed. Some patients can produce a long panel to hang; one patient designed a festival panel that she donated to her church.

The silk is pinned onto frames, we find and outline a design, then paint and blend the colours. This is a much longer process than painting scarves. We work out a design and then pipe on an outline, which restricts where the colour stays. The easiest way is to put the gutta in a pipette with a nib and pipe the outline of the design. There is another process where you could paint the silk with anti-fusion and then just use it as you would a canvas if you were painting. This requires greater artistic skill.

Box 7.2 Silk painting

Painting a silk scarf

Materials

   Silk scarf

   Steam fix dyes

   Small containers to put the dye in

   Plastic droppers

   Table or rock salt (optional)

   Steamer or saucepan and colander

   Rubber gloves

   Disposable plastic aprons

   Masking tape or sellotape

Process

We use 140cm × 50cm scarves; these have been more popular than square ones. The weight of the silk is pongee 5. We purchase all our silk painting materials from Rainbow Silks. They carry a very large stock and are always helpful if you have any problems with the craft. We advise choosing no more than three colours.

First prepare the area you are going to use by covering with plastic. We have found thin disposable aprons ideal for this. Lay the apron out on the surface and secure with small pieces of tape. Place the scarf on the plastic and spray it with water. The scarf needs to be wet all over but not soaked. Then, pleat the scarf so that it stands up in peaks. You do not want the scarf to be flat on the work surface or the dyes will not be able to flow properly. Place a dropper into the dye, squeeze the bulb to draw up the dye and then slowly drip the dye over the scarf working with one colour at a time, working your way up the length of the scarf leaving areas of white scarf still showing then drip on the second colour in the same way and then the third. You should see the dyes running into each other, forming other colours. You can now sprinkle the scarf generously with salt if you wish; leave for five minutes. This draws out some of the dye, forming interesting patterns on the scarf.

After the five minutes, the scarf can be gathered gently together and put in the basket of the steamer. We use plastic vegetable steamers that are suitable for the microwave. A small amount of water is put in the base of the steam bowl. It is very important that the water does not come above the base of the basket, and that the scarf does not sit in a pool of water. Place the lid on the container and put in microwave on full power for seven minutes. If you do not have a steamer you can get the same effect by placing the scarf in a colander with a lid on it over a saucepan of boiling water. Remove scarf from container taking care as it will be hot and rinse the scarf in lukewarm water until it runs clear, squeeze out excess moisture and iron.

You can easily do this craft with very few dyes as they are all intermixable. I would advise having the primary colours and two or three more. We use Dupont steam fix dyes which are available in 50ml and 250ml bottles.

Silk painting

Basic equipment and materials for silk painting

Silk

Selection of dyes

Plastic pipette with nib (we use size 0.8)

Masking tape

Silk pins

Palette

Dropper for transferring dyes to palette

Pencil

Paintbrushes

Frame

Gutta

Hairdryer – used for drying gutta and dyes

Water pots

Frames

Process

Cover the edge of the frame with masking tape before starting, to prevent dye penetrating the wood and staining the next piece of work. Remove the tape after each painting is finished, replacing it with new tape. Stretch the silk tightly over the frame with silk pins so that the design can be transferred. Place the template underneath the silk and secure with small pieces of tape; draw the design with a soft 2B pencil then remove the paper from behind the silk.

Gently squeeze the full pipette of gutta and apply it to the surface of silk following the traced design, making sure that there are no breaks in the line.

When the gutta is dry, you can start painting the silk. Put a small amount of dye on your brush and place point of brush on the silk and you will find the dye will spread quickly across the surface of the silk avoiding the need of too many brushstrokes. If there is not enough dye to fill the area, apply some more immediately until you are happy with the results. If you have applied too much dye to the area and there is a puddle, the excess can be removed using a cotton bud. All dyes are intermixable so shading and exciting results can soon be achieved with practice. If you wish you start something small to gain confidence, embroidery frames are ideal to stretch the silk on. If you are happy with

Over the time that I have been doing craft, I have built up folders of templates. If patients are nervous about doing their own design, they can go through the folders and choose a template. We enlarge or reduce it and transfer it onto the silk. Alternatively, if they are good at drawing with a pencil, patients will transfer the design onto the silk themselves. Most manage the guttaring themselves, but if they are not well enough or do not have enough strength in their hands, I will do it for them.

The painting is done using the same steam-fix dyes but fixing is a totally different process. When it comes to steaming to fix the colours, you can't put a silk painting into a microwave because, unlike the scarves whose colours are intended to run into each other, a silk picture or panel needs to stay as it was painted. Therefore, we roll them on a roller with another piece of fabric so the silk does not touch the other pieces of silk; we steam it for about an hour in a specialist steamer.

Assistance and 'doing it myself'

Where people have limited physical ability, either I or volunteers help. One lady I have been working with has very limited mobility but she has been turning out the most amazing silk paintings with a paint brush on silk. We stretch the silk onto a frame so that it is taut and she brushes the dye on.

We respond naturally as people's capacity to carry out particular tasks changes. One man's mobility became less and less as he was doing picture frames, but he would always direct where he wanted a particular colour. We would never make that decision. I would never put my ideas forward; I would not say what the colours should be or where a tile should be placed. Sometimes, patients have actually said: 'Can you help me; I'm struggling with this', and of course we will advise and give all the help we can. However, at the end of the day it is their decision, their work. It would be very easy to take over the choice of colours; to say that they are not right just because they are not to our taste.

Jack, the union official with motor neurone disease, did come to a point where he said: 'I now need help': then obviously we gave it on a one-to-one basis. When he was making the coffee table, one of us would work with him all the time, because otherwise he could not continue with the project. He could still speak and he had a great sense of humour; he would still say where he wanted something put, and he designed the Newcastle United table for his wife. We obviously had to do the cutting of the tiles and eventually it came to the point where we had to stick them on for him – but under his direction.

Other craft work and projects

We talk over with patients and show them the possibilities of other craft work. An important and popular activity is painting on glass, porcelain and ceramics (see Box 7.3 for details). This requires care and capacity to do detailed work, which some patients are unable to achieve. However, as with other crafts, it is possible to help or to work on behalf of the patient.

The main features of sugar craft are how to marzipan and sugar-paste a cake, how to make sugar flowers and how to sculpture in sugar. It is unusual for either women or men patients to have done sugar craft before; often they are not even aware of the term. However, they find it interesting once you show them what it involves. It is useful if it has a connection with a time of the year or an event in a patient's life, such as a birthday. We always do it at Christmas and Easter, and normally at one other time during the year I will introduce it.

Other craft work that we do occasionally when there is a demand or need, is card making. We collect old cards which can be recycled to make new designs. You can readily buy aperture card blanks and various attractive stick-on items and lettering. Simple designs work best. These can be sold to raise funds, but many patients also like to send their own hand-made cards.

We have done a number of shared craft projects, which can involve large numbers of patients, and Tasker in Chapter 9 describes the process of building up projects to gain patients' and others' involvement. However, within a con-tinuous day unit group, we have introduced a range of collage-making activities that can involve several patients working together. We ask people to bring in pieces of broken or unused materials in a particular category. For example, spare jewellery or watches seem to be widely available; ideas are only limited by the group's imagination. The groups work to sort them out, and then contribute to sticking them into a design. For example, we have collages of candles, star and a Christmas tree in jewellery, and a large candle in clock and watch parts.

Another recent project used our experience of mosaic work. We designed continuous panels of mosaic to go round the low walls of a pond in the hospice garden; they were linked together by a thread of mirror tiles representing a river round the walls. We divided the design into panels, and set up tables in the garden. Patients, carers, visitors, staff, volunteers and anyone who came into the hospice – including some important people visiting the chief executive – was

Box 7.3 Painting on glass or ceramics

Painting on glass
Materials

    Glass paints

    Range of small paint brushes

    Clear glass plates, bases, tumblers etc.

    Masking tape

    Range of pre-drawn design templates if required. These are available in a wide choice of subjects from Search Press and can be enlarged or reduced on a photocopier to fit the piece of glass

    Cotton buds

    Outliner – this is an acrylic paste piped straight from the tube like icing a cake. Outliner comes in a range of colours but I have found the most popular to be gold and black

Process

Having chosen your design attach it to the glass with a small piece of tape; if you are working on a plate the template should be placed underneath so that the design is visible. If it is a vase or tumbler etc. the template should be placed on the inside showing the design through the side of the glass. You can of course draw your own design on to paper and attach in the same way. If you are doing your own design, I would advise not to draw anything with very fine lines as the nozzle on the outliner tubes will not be suitable.

    Gently squeeze the tube of outliner following the design showing through the glass. After completing a section of the piping always clear the excess outliner off the nozzle. When finished allow the outliner to dry thoroughly; this can be speeded up with a hairdryer.

    Stir the paint well and using one colour at a time apply to one section at a time on the glass with a brush, first working the paint into the outlined edges of your design and then filling in the sections in between. Try to avoid too much brushing of the paint as this forms streaks. You get a better effect if you apply the paint with the tip of the brush gently filling the area with colour. All the colours are intermixable so with a bit of practice you can achieve some lovely results with blending one colour into another. This is very effective when painting flowers. If you are painting a plate you can leave it flat on the table. If you are working on a vase or tumbler it is advisable to lay the piece down on a towel or support to avoid the paint running down the side. Any excess paint can be removed with a cotton bud. When the piece is finished, allow it to air dry for 24 hours before fixing. This is usually done in a domestic oven; times and temperature will vary depending on the paints you choose. We use Deka Crystal transparent water-based paints. I would not recommend solvent-based glass paints as they give off a very strong odour.

IKEA carry a very good and inexpensive range of glass plates and vases which can be used for this craft. Their straight-sided glass tumblers are perfect for the transparent paints and for placing a tea light inside.

Painting ceramics
Materials

Ceramic paints (we use Pebeo 160)

Small paint brushes

Outliner – this is an acrylic paste piped straight from the tube. Outliner comes in a range of colours but I have found gold and black to be the most popular

Range of templates that can be enlarged or reduced on a photocopier

Cotton buds

Carbon paper

Pencil

Masking tape

Process

Choose your template; make sure it is the right size for the piece you are going to be working on. Transfer the design on to the china: with a small piece of masking tape, attach the template where you want the design to be and put a piece of carbon paper underneath, pencil over the design making sure you do not miss anything. It is best to use a coloured pencil to make it easier to see where you have drawn. Remove the tape and paper and your design will be transferred to the china. Do not worry if the carbon has smudged because it is easily removed when you have finished outlining.

Gently squeeze the tube of outliner following the design. After completing each section clear the excess outliner off the nozzle. When finished, allow to dry thoroughly. This can speeded up with a hairdryer.

To commence painting, stir the paint thoroughly and apply to one section at a time, first brushing the paint into the edges of the outliner and then filling the area with paint. Try to avoid too much brushing as this forms streaks. It is better to apply the paint with the tip of your brush filling the area with paint.

Allow to air dry for at least 24 hours and then fix in a domestic oven. With Pebeo 160 you place the painted piece in a cold oven and set it for 150–160°C. When the oven has reached the required temperature, you time it for 35 minutes then turn the oven off, leaving the piece inside until the oven has cooled down.

asked to help. There was a lot of camaraderie, and some people spent hours fitting little pieces of tile in to the designs. These were applied to the walls and then grouted and polished exactly as the mirrors and tables are dealt with.

Case study: Tom

Tom was a man in his forties who had been in the police force for 30 years and had been part of the flying squad. He was admitted to the inpatient unit for drug control and to manage his fits having been diagnosed six months earlier with a brain tumour. The ward staff asked for a member of the arts team to talk with him about attending the day unit; initially he was not interested and felt it would be not be for him, thinking it would be full of old people. We felt that the best approach was to take to him some samples of craft that are easily achieved on the ward either at the bedside or in bed. He very quickly became involved in working with clay. His eyesight was failing and he enjoyed the tactile feel of the clay. With a finished sample in front of him that he could keep on looking at and touching, he managed to produce the first of his many pottery elephants. His wife could not believe that he so quickly became engrossed in the activity and, since we were working regularly with him in his room, she managed to leave the ward and take a much-needed break; previously, Tom did not want her to leave the room.

After the initial contact with Tom, his wife brought him to look around the day unit and talk about the other activities. We could see that he was enjoying the thought of more craft work and was already planning other pieces of work for specific members of the family including his wife and the four children.

After his two weeks on the ward and several visits to the day unit as an inpatient, Tom was discharged. He told his wife he did not want to go home as he felt comfortable and safe and was enjoying himself. A referral was made by the ward staff for him to attend the day unit twice a week.

On his first visit to the day unit, Tom had already decided what his first piece of craft was to be and over the course of the next few weeks he produced another ten pottery elephants, which he glazed in an assortment of colours, for particular members of his family. He then went on to make mosaic mirrors; these he produced in particular colours for family members: often he would choose the colours of the football team they supported. This was very apparent when he was making them for his children.

Tom was always willing and excited in trying a new craft and was very soon producing dozens of silk scarves that he was giving away as presents. He found this craft very easy as he was having trouble with limited mobility in one hand and also his eyesight was failing. As usual he always knew what colours he wanted to use and would come into the centre with a list of who he wanted to make the next piece for. He looked forward to his visits to the centre and would always make sure that if his hospital appointment coincided with one of his day unit days he would be brought on to the day unit even if it meant he only got half a day. His wife was amazed at the enthusiasm he had for craft as he had never done any before and the only thing he had been involved in was amateur dramatics and occasionally writing poetry.

Tom was a sociable man with a great sense of humour. Because of his experience of limited eyesight and mobility, he was very supportive to other patients, encouraging them to have a go. He was very proud of telling them what he had managed to make. His wife always said that when he returned from the unit with another piece of work, he could not wait to show the family. She said that he enjoyed everything at St Christopher's and she is sure that his visits and the pieces that they were making kept him going. It gave him belief in himself and something to look forward to.

Tom's last piece of work was to be a mosaic clock. It was his idea that the piece was to be made in green and white glass mosaic tiles with his and his wife and children's names arranged in a crossword style around the clock. The mosaic also included a white dove and the ichthus. He had given a great deal of thought to the design he wanted on the piece and was adamant as to where the names and designs were to go. I admired his strength and determination to, in what were to be the last few weeks of his life, make this piece for his family. He had not told any of them that he was working on the clock as he wanted it to be a surprise but unfortunately he died just before the piece was finished. He had managed to attach all the tiles in place, despite being so ill. He had asked me whether, if he did not manage to finish it, I would complete it for him and give it to his wife. It was an emotional time for her receiving the clock as she had no idea that he had been working on it and kept it a secret. She and many other members of the family have some amazing pieces of work to cherish that Tom made in the six months that he was under St Christopher's care. I would like to think that the introduction he had to the day unit and craft work gave Tom a purpose in life, not only enjoying and producing a range of beautiful pieces of work but also knowing that they would be cherished by his family.

Conclusion

Craft work offers a range of achievable objectives, which can be stimulating and enjoyable to patients, and many other people, and quickly produces attractive results. People can develop as craftspeople and can also join together to make interesting joint projects, which are very engaging. As the basis for creative activities in a continuing day care programme, or at the bedside in people's homes or as an inpatient, they can generate a lot of interaction between patients, families and carers and produce worthwhile gifts for patients to 'give something back' rather than just feel a burden to their families and carers.

Equipment and resources

The main specialist piece of equipment we have is the steamer for rolled silk panels.

For mosaic work we buy simple plain picture frames, mirrors and coffee tables from IKEA. The mosaic tiles come from Mosaic Workshop in London; they have a shop and workshop and send tiles, grout etc. out by mail order all over the country. They have a website and a very comprehensive catalogue.

For silk painting templates, we mainly use books of designs from Search Press; there is very wide choice of flowers, Egyptian, Chinese, Japanese and Art Nouveau designs, and many more. Flowers or animals are always popular as are designs for children.

Card making and other similar craft resources can be bought from most stationers, such as IKEA, Lakeland and W.H. Smith's. The materials we purchase are from Craft Creations.

9 Digital Arts

Marion Tasker

Introducing digital art

At St Christopher's Hospice a long tradition exists of offering psychosocial and spiritual care by providing opportunities for patients to express themselves in a creative way, through painting and drawing, pottery, crafts, gardening and horticultural therapy, reminiscence, creative writing and art or music therapy. We do this by working with patients and their families in a variety of settings, expanding from a base in the day unit to work on the inpatient unit wards and out into the community, visiting in their homes patients who are unable or do not wish to attend the hospice. Using digital equipment can offer people a new way of exploring their feelings and telling their stories, or of producing art in a very different way from our traditional offerings through photography, video, poetry, music. Although initially the words 'digital art' seem daunting, once you embark on a journey past the technology you find a new realm of expression.

When I began to facilitate a digital art group in the Creative Living Centre it was a task in itself, but to run one that was to replace a well-established and popular gardening group/'club' made the task seem even more difficult. I found myself standing in front of a group of patients explaining that I was going to introduce them to a new medium. The response as expected was less than enthusiastic. I tried to sound encouraging and sell the idea to them but of course they saw through me. I left work that day feeling discouraged and the only thing that had developed substantially was my insecurity and feeling that I didn't have the skills to run any group.

I spent the week thinking how I could swing things around and get people involved. We didn't have a huge amount of equipment: three digital cameras, two mini-tripods and two laptops and I had a group of (on average) ten people.

There were also the limitations of patient mobility to consider. Several of my group were in wheelchairs and one woman in particular was shaky with Parkinson's disease. How could I ensure that no one was excluded?

I tried to devise a project that would incorporate all different kinds of media, thinking that if digital photography were used alongside painting it wouldn't seem so alien and the technical side of it wouldn't intimidate people so much. The 'digital' mixed media collage tree came about. This was created on a piece of medium density fibreboard (MDF) board cut to a size of eight feet long by four feet wide. We painted the board with white emulsion. I then asked the members of the group who were able to go out and photograph a tree in the garden. They came back, we looked at the photographs and chose one that we thought would work well as an image. I then talked to them about how old masters sometimes used a device called the *camera lucida* to project an image onto their canvas to draw from. I linked this old method to the new tools we had and projected the photograph of the tree onto the MDF board. They then drew around it. The following week, everyone in the group became involved and used the digital cameras. Even those people whose mobility was limited were able to do table-top photography. I brought in as many pieces of bark for them to photograph as I could: we even had some small specimens of wildlife crawling across the tables. We used small sponges to paint a sky background in acrylic paint. We then printed all the bark and leaf photographs, cut or tore them into small pieces and then stuck them onto the board to complete the collage. The group produced a beautiful piece of art. In fact to my surprise as we held up the finished piece everyone spontaneously clapped, thrilled with what they achieved. Not only did we now have a piece of work for display in the hospice but I showed the group what they had accomplished and how we could photograph the work and print off copies that could be made into cards as a memento of their work.

Developing digital art

I had proved to myself that it could work; however this was only the beginning. Each week I try to come up with interesting projects that the group will find challenging enough to engage them and stretch them. This clearly is not art therapy but does have therapeutic value. The group has evolved over the past couple of years as a sharing group. When asked if they would like to develop individual projects, on the whole they have declined. They prefer to have a shared experience, each taking on a complementary role. Some members prefer photography, while others have found a more traditional medium, but we manage to mix the two successfully.

Our approach is to develop a shared experience, so that people feel they are trying something new in the knowledge that they are supported and encouraged by those around them. Each project we have worked on has brought about discussions that may not come about in another setting. Symptoms, fears, worries and feelings of isolation are aired in discussion, as well as feelings of joy and relief when something positive is achieved. Despite at times being obviously tired and in pain, the group somehow carry each other along with a combined energy that is not visible but is definitely there. I have on several occasions seen how a member of the group arrived in the morning very low in mood, looking weak and expressing only a desire to watch in a chair, by the end of the morning is actively involved, animated and smiling.

Digital media might be used in many different ways with people of different abilities and motilities. Age is immaterial, all that is needed is a willingness to experiment and have a go. Often, people are delighted at the results and thrilled at seeing the work; particularly when family members reinforce the feelings of empowerment.

There has been certain pleasure in being able to surprise their computer-literate grandchildren by showing off some of their digital photographs and also being able to give them their email address.

Responses

Prior to running the group I had used both digital stills cameras and digital video cameras with patients on a one-to-one basis and also in conjunction with family members.

Much of this work has been to enable patients to leave a legacy for their family. Or, as in the case of one man I worked with, to enable his young daughter to know 'who he is'. It is a human need to be remembered, to have made our mark in however small a way. This may be a public mark, for immediate family or as an individual. It enables people to feel that they have in some way contributed, been heard and/or acknowledged.

People's lives can be a mix of challenging, hard and difficult emotional times. Some people through their personal experience may be more confident and forthcoming in sharing those experiences and, as they begin to build in confidence and relate these important memories, others in the group may start to think that their life is less interesting and become reluctant to participate verbally, preferring to be a listener. It is important to encourage the sharing of memories and give each person in the group time to speak and make them feel valued.

A had been part of the reminiscence group and had a lot to share. However, often it became difficult to facilitate this in a way that would be valuable for him without making other members of the group feel that they hadn't the opportunity to speak. He would often linger on specific times that he wanted to expand on, regardless of the theme that the group might have been following. This was compounded by slight hearing loss. I asked A if he would like the time to work on a one-to-one basis to give him more time to explore his memories. He seemed delighted at the proposal and we worked for six weeks, talking about the important times that he wanted to record in some way.

We made a video of his memories that he was extremely pleased with and he later rejoined the group able to listen to and enjoy others' experiences. The advantage of digital media is that it is immediate. Patients in palliative care often do not have the luxury of time; time is but a moment and that moment needs to be recognised and embraced.

Case study: a fashion show project conceived by women attending the Creative Living Centre

The starting point: listening

We have found that user-led projects are the most successful since the user self-direction makes them rewarding and relevant to those involved. They offer ways in which we can specifically meet the needs for self-fulfilment of people who access hospice services. In their artistic outcomes, they may also be stimulating and inspiring for observers, and if appropriately recorded and displayed, may continue to make a contribution to people's motivation and progress over a long period. This particular project seemed to encompass all of these elements and continues to inspire those who are able to hear about it. It is also important to note its achievability. Often when we read about a project that others have worked on, we think: 'Oh, I couldn't possibly do that; we don't have the resources', yet this project cost very little financially and was contained in a structured way so that time could be well managed.

The key is to identify whether we are working with individuals or groups, a desire or need for expression that we can extract, draw out and nurture so that they can reach their potential and realise their dreams or even go beyond. It is important to acknowledge ideas so that they do not go unnoticed, lie dormant or stagnate.

I had been working on a short piece of work with one of the women that attend the day unit on a Thursday. It involved compiling a series of selected photographs in the form of a movie that was to be shown at her memorial service. The project wasn't just about the putting together of the photographs but about her journey as a whole. As with much of the work I have been involved with, the process that takes place before the completion of video or photography is of huge significance, often more so than the final piece. On the surface, she seemed to be a woman in tune with and in control of the way she was feeling and the effect her illness was having on her and those close to her.

However, it began to emerge that there was underlying turmoil, anger and fear. Overloading herself with tasks to realise before her death seemed to be her way of facing and yet avoiding aspects that were too difficult to address. Her faith was paramount and she was calling on this to give her both strength and also answers she needed about why she was facing her own death at such a young age, before she had had a chance to achieve many of her hopes and desires as a woman.

We spent some time discussing the length of the piece, the music to be used and the relevance of each picture selected and how it documented parts of her life. We also spent time discussing how it might be for the people that she had decided would be going to see the compilation. At the time, she seemed very angry at the way that the closest members of her family and friends were reacting to her and her illness.

The final picture of the sequence was to be special and was to represent how she was now. In her words: 'I don't want to be remembered by some dodgy photograph that my mum or sister dig out from the eighties.' Again, she was expressing a need to be in control of her destiny and life right to the end.

We were now at the point where we needed this special picture. She wanted to be seen in an outfit that represented her personality, her culture, and her heritage. She mentioned that she planned to write to the Willow Foundation (www.willowfoundation.org.uk/home.shtml). They organise and finance special days for people under the age of 40 years who are terminally ill. Her request was that she be able to work for a day with a fashion designer to create an outfit, according to her needs and specifications.

Several other women joined the discussion and it became clear that they, too, were having a similar experience in trying to buy clothes that would make them feel comfortable and beautiful. They were all going through the many adverse affects of their illness and treatment. Among these were tiredness (often they didn't have the energy to trawl the shops for something that would fit and look nice), sickness, fluctuating weight, weight loss and weight gain, hair loss and oedemic arms and legs.

Listening as they talked, I started to think that maybe I could ring up the London College of Fashion (LCF) to see if students would be interested in coming to work on a project with us. I mentioned the idea and the women agreed that we should see if we would get any response.

Developing partnerships in the project

To contact the relevant professional/students we needed, I rang LCF and spoke to several different departments before I eventually got put through to Laurie Cansfield of VITAL (Volunteering in the Arts for London). He felt the idea was attainable; VITAL had been involved in similar projects. I completed various forms relating to our requirements of potential volunteers, and this was then posted on their website bulletin board.

Two weeks went by and I got a call from Chris Scottburrows, volunteer coordinator for VITAL. He had four volunteers that he would like to bring along to meet with us. We set a date.

We were extremely lucky to have a response from skilled and relevant volunteers (see the appendix to this chapter). Caterina had worked with women with disability and so had an insight into creating comfortable, beautiful garments for individual body shapes. Peter came with both his skills as a technician and his personal experience of illness which enabled him to be sensitive to the hospice environment. Natalie, Daniella and Manjinder came with a freshness and enthusiasm.

Martyn, a personal friend, had been interrogated by me because I wanted him on the project too. I needed to know he really understood what we needed. I wanted him to be involved because I didn't want the complication of using other professional photographers where copyright might become an issue. He had worked in the fashion industry, covered London Fashion Week and photographed at many high-profile events.

Prior to introducing the volunteers to the women, we discussed with them St Christopher's as an organisation and on the role of creative arts in our work. We also reviewed with them what they might wish to get from their part in this collaboration. They also had an opportunity to ask any questions about what might be involved and express any concerns or worries that they might have about working in the hospice.

The project

We all met and discussed the individual needs and aspirations that the women and volunteers had for the project. The volunteers were keen not to be seen as a dressmaking service and wanted it to be an experience where we all worked together as a team.

We set a plan to run over the next six weeks. We would meet each Thursday. At this point we didn't discuss the budget.

The women wanted to make it clear that although they were totally committed to the project there might be weeks when they would be unable to attend because of hospital appointments or illness; that was discussed too.

The plan was as follows:

Week 1: Talking about ideas.

Week 2: The volunteers brought in examples of work and portfolios.

Week 3: Sketching, colour, fabric.

Week 4: Starting to cut toiles, fitting.

Week 5: Visit to the London College of Fashion.

Week 6: The show.

We then looked at potential costs.

- *Materials*: Some fabric was given by the LCF from their storeroom, some was bought by the women themselves and some was financed by the hospice arts budget (this amounted to less than £150). A sewing machine was loaned to us. Pencils, paper, sketchpads we had already.

- *Space*: A vital commodity to provide a secure base for the duration of the project.

- *Time*: The volunteers gave a great deal of time to the project apart from the Thursdays that they attended St Christopher's. Caterina and Peter searched for fabric. They also spent time cutting out and making up the final garments with the help of Manjinder and one of her fellow students, who machined up the dresses. All of them also had end of year shows and Manjinder was graduating! So their dedication to the project cannot go unrecognised.

- *Other costs*:

  ◦ The volunteers' travel expenses were met through the hospice personnel budget.

  ◦ The college provided lunch when we went on our trip to LCF. We travelled by the hospice mini-bus driven by one of our volunteer drivers; this had to be booked in advance to ensure that they were available.

  ◦ The day of the show, we spent a little on tea and cakes for visitors.

A lot of my time was spent on making sure everyone was happy with the designs, a display background for the fashion show, the venue for the show booked (the hospice chapel), people invited, photography arranged, leaflets, posters designed and arranged. I also worked to keep momentum and enthusiasm going.

The downs

There were times that the project members became disheartened because of a feeling that their vision wasn't being realised and that maybe some of their ideas were simply not possible, given the time and resources that we had. Material was more difficult to get than I had expected: where have all the fabric shops gone?

One of the lecturers produced some material for a jacket to the response from the designer: 'It's hideous! I'll wear it for the show but I wouldn't be seen dead in it afterwards.' Not quite the reaction we hoped for, but I must admit she was right and so Caterina searched and managed to find something much more suitable, just days before the show. Each woman had at least one week that they were unable to attend. Sometimes students were late, lecturers didn't turn up and I dashed around fretting.

As with life there were events that were out of our control and the London bombings on 7 July 2006 affected us both psychologically and practically: some of the volunteers had to find ways to get home and get in touch with relatives who might be worried. Much of that Thursday was spent making sure they were able to find alternative ways back home.

The trip to the college

This was my first experience of organising a trip. First, we needed to make sure we had a nurse with us and that had delayed the trip by a week. However, the original week we had planned was the week of the bombing so somehow, as throughout the project, we felt that events played out in a very special way. LCF is in an old Victorian building with eight floors and no lift or disabled access. We fortunately only needed to get up to first floor and we could base ourselves in the staff room on ground level. Toilets were on ground level too. We booked the mini-bus and volunteer driver well in advance and all kept fingers crossed that the women would be well enough to make the trip. They were, although one woman had a hospital appointment and so couldn't come so we made sure we had everything we needed from her to cut out her material and start to machine her dress. Although the day was tiring it was also exciting. Because we were now on the final stretch of the project, the adrenaline was flowing and stress levels of the volunteers rising. The project members remained calm.

The day of the show

The project members had compiled descriptions of their outfits and inspiration. They also chose some suitable music to be played during the show which reflected their feelings and emotions regarding both themselves and their part in the project. Martyn arrived to spend the day with us. He looked around the garden to source the best backgrounds to complement the colours of the garments and put the women at their ease as they posed for their special photographs. He used a digital SLR camera, which enabled him to download all the images that he had taken onto our computer on the same day. This ensured that the women had sole ownership of any photographs taken and knew that they were in control of where those images were shown. I was particularly conscious of the fact that there had been interest from the national press and there was a danger that the women would start to feel that they were losing control of the project. There was an air of calmness (from the women), an air of panic (from me) and an air of angst and slight disbelief that it was all happening today (from the volunteers). I had taken a chance and double-booked a band for the chapel just before the girls were supposed to go on and was hoping that it would all work. It did: the band set the stage for the event because the music drew people from different parts of the building; some because it had reminded them of the fashion event; others came out of curiosity.

We were all still in the project base minutes before we were to come on, making last minute adjustments to the outfits, college students were taking photographs and I was quickly running through where they were to walk once in the chapel, because we hadn't had the luxury of a rehearsal!

I was clinging to a notebook, which was acting a prop for me as I was becoming increasingly nervous about how I was going to introduce the event.

We all made our way along the corridor to the chapel; the music from the band beckoned us forth. I ushered the girls into the little room at the side of the chapel and then peered around the door to see who had come. I was just amazed the chapel was full.

As I nervously faced the crowd, I felt a wave of warmth and love that made me feel at ease and extremely proud to have been able to work with such a supporting team of professionals without whom I could never manage a venture like this.

I spoke a little about the project as did Peter and Caterina. We showed slides of the work in progress with 'Something so Strong' as the backing track, and then the women came in one by one. All of them were iconic, since each was different, very individual. The incredible strength that shone through was amazing and inspirational. It is difficult to express in words here exactly what happened and how special it was. It was almost spiritual in nature and as such the written word is, on this occasion, inadequate.

The significance for people involved

The question most asked given the success of this project is would we be doing it again. I don't think we could. It was special because of the people that came together in that moment in time. It was special because it was user-led. It was special because it was a true collaboration between people that wouldn't ordinarily come into contact with each other. It was special because everyone took something unique away from the experience.

All of the women said that on the day it had felt marvellous to be centre of attention, to be admired, to be photographed, to feel proud. They all felt that they had been appreciated as people and not patients. Sometimes it seems the person becomes the illness and is only recognised by their illness. Even, at times, they have been introduced as, 'This is Joan who has breast cancer', as if it was the disease that defined the person.

For one woman, the experience for her was how she imagined it would be if she were the bride walking down the aisle, realising that this maybe the closest she would get to have that experience. Two of the women wore their dresses at their own funerals and their families displayed those very special photographs just as they had wished. For the family members that attended it was a feeling of pride and admiration.

One of the women wrote the following on the evening of the show: 'We were beautiful today and I was proud to belong to a special team. I came home realising that I can be creative and imaginative if I put my mind to it.'

People in the audience were also affected. There was a significant response after the show and below are some observations and feelings that people were left with.

> I so enjoyed last week's fashion show and learning about all your hard work in creating your beautiful outfits. You all looked so lovely and I think you really achieved what you set out to do – to show us who you are as people, as women as whole human beings with an inner and outer beauty. I hope you all enjoyed the show as much as we did watching it.
>
> I have thought about you all a lot since last week and wanted you to know how lovely it was to see you smiling, confident and proud of who you are. Thank you for letting us see your marvellous creations and for being who you are.

The women's faces said it all. They worked hard, and turned a page of energy and freshness, also sexuality for themselves that they thought was lost.

I feel we need to be sensitive to the impact of such projects on both the patients, the staff members and also the volunteers. When one becomes involved in a project that demands so much energy both physical and psychological it can play a significant role in your life for the duration and when the end of that project arrives one has to address that for some a small void might be left. While it will be easy for one person to move forward and embark on the next stage of their journey, becoming quickly involved in the other activities or experiences available to them, for another it might be a time of reflection and maybe a feeling of 'So what do I do now?'; a time when they might feel low, a time when the events of the previous weeks may have forced them to face their own reality. So it is important to support them through this period at their own pace, yet caringly guide them forward; to keep the essence of the experience with them as a tool to face the challenges ahead.

Case study: 'Fat black kid in the corner'

One of my first referrals from the hospice home care team was for a young man; Paul, who was blind and bedbound, living in a nursing home. Despite regular visits from his family, he felt very isolated and desperate to have his voice heard. He would often tell me how lone he felt and staff at the nursing home would tell how he would ring up family members at all hours feeling anxious and afraid. This was voiced in his poetry. He had a lot to say. Much of what he wanted recorded was about his body image and sense of self.

Paul relayed to me many powerful pieces of work. He was keen to have his work read and commented upon by others and so I am happy to publish it here. It was empowering for him to have his work recorded on video and shown to others. Indeed, when it was published on the Rosetta Life website a connection was made with another patient at Greenwich and Bexley Hospice and that eased Paul's feeling of being alone. There were several communications where comments from other hospice users would be placed on the Rosetta website and which I would in turn read to Paul. He seemed genuinely amazed and delighted at the response from readers of his work. I feel that he felt a need to express his feelings and although the accolade of a positive response was well received it was the actual spewing of the words from his very being that was so cathartic. He continued to work with me once a week over a period of three months until he died.

Fat black kid in the corner

I've been that fat
Black kid in the corner
All my life
And I could handle it
Now
I'm that fat black kid in the corner
Who can't see
Whose hand is always held out
Always in need
See like
When you're that fat black kid in the corner
You learn not to need too much
You learn how to get by
If a girl is willing to go with you
Great guns
But if she suddenly changes her mind
No hardship
Because I've always been a big man
I've always been careful
I'm no rapist
I'm no man who bullies his woman
Although sometimes I wish I could
'Cause I see them leave me
For other guys who hurt them
But
I'm the fat black kid in the corner
So I watch and philosophise
And stand on the side
Now I'm blind
So how comes
I didn't grab one
When I could see
Like all my friends told me to
Grab her she do alright
She really likes you
You'll be in there son
But now I'm blind
Where will I be well in?
I'm without of everything

Lots of my friends
I've lost their telephone numbers
Because I've lost my pieces of paper
Which I used to write them down on
And there's no one there to search out
All those intimate things for me any more
Because I was the fat black kid in the corner
I did all these things myself
I knew how to repair things
I knew how to make things work
Because that way
Wouldn't have to beg anyone anything
I would always stand in the corner
And get by
By, By
Getting by
Bye, Bye
Getting by
The kid in the corner
Who can't get by
Who's blind
Who wants to cry

The End

Paul Moore, May 2005

Case study: portraits: our body image 'face to face'

It has been interesting to me to find that the theme that I am most interested in – that of self-image is the one that I have been slightly hesitant about introducing because of the implications of discussion with those whose body image has very often changed dramatically – has been the one that people have engaged in very quickly. I do my best to evade the wrong side of the camera, yet I find that members of the group very keen to be recorded in a similar way to the women who were involved in the fashion project.

I introduced to the group the idea of portraiture in different media. I have found that at the outset of any project it is often the group discussion prior that creates a solid foundation for our imaginations to fly. We sat around a table and one by one I invited members of the group to talk about if they felt comfortable, about how they would like to portray the essence of their being to the world. As part of this sharing of experiences, one man talked about the importance of time and how he always wanted to be able to see a clock or have a watch on. He talked about his time as a foreman; how punctuality was instilled in his workers: clocking on and clocking off; how none of us should waste a moment. He would want this to be reflected in his portrait: he enjoyed time.

Another member of the group cut into the discussion saying: 'Of course, time can work against you; my time is running out.'

One member of the group who attends each week in beautiful African gowns is particularly keen to have her image recorded. I asked her about this and the dresses that she wears and her response was: 'I have a wardrobe of them and I must wear them all before I die.' She very openly looks at the photographs that we have started to take each week, not so interested in the quality of the photograph, the lighting and the clarity but more concerned with the character. It is as if she is taken out of herself and able to reflect on the person before her, remarking how her face has changed its shape and expression and going on to disclose feelings of physical discomfort and then deeper into fears: 'I don't know what is going to happen to me.'

We spent the afternoon taking the portraits. My role was purely encouragement, very little technical intervention. There was a lot of playful banter that enabled everyone to be relaxed and play to the camera. The following week I projected the portraits onto a screen for everyone to see; the best were chosen. As soon as each person had selected their favourite picture, we started to talk as a group about what the photograph said to us; did it match our discussions prior to the photo shoot? As people began to talk about their reaction to the portraits, I asked individuals one by one for a word, phrase or sentence that would describe their personal response to the image before them. Collectively we produced some poignant and poetic writing. It is interesting to note that in previous sessions when I had suggested we do some creative writing as a group there had been some hesitancy, many saying they couldn't write yet somehow the portraits prompted a response; now the words started to flow in a beautifully explicit way.

We printed the poems off with the portraits and displayed them along a hospice corridor. Families, members of staff and other visitors to the hospice have commented that each portrait is so personal and individual the group really managed to capture an element of their character. Family members have been pleased to have a portrait that in many ways is rather unconventional, together with a small piece of writing expressing a brief moment in time. Considering many of the group had never picked up a camera before the quality of the work and individuality of each piece is quite incredible.

Conclusion

Our hope is that in writing about these projects others will be inspired enough to develop their own ideas within their own organisations. However, it would be superficial if I only wrote of the positive aspects of the project; there were of course aspects that push us to face the stark fact that all of these people have a terminal diagnosis.

Every one of these projects required a huge investment of time and energy to keep the momentum going.

What was the importance of these projects, beyond that of image, hope, recognition, acknowledgement? I observed for my part several overt changes that the women went through who were involved in the fashion show. One had been on the inpatient wards for some weeks and had been reluctant to come to the day unit. She sat quietly on the perimeter. Observing but not engaging. I was aware that she had been angry and unhappy on the ward and I was keen for her to find something that she could become involved with that would be challenging, but fulfilling, that might give her the opportunity talk and share, with others that were going through similar experience. A group project like this can facilitate discussion at a deeper level. By the end of the project a change had happened. The words I would have used to describe her before might have been withdrawn, sad, angry, hostile, defensive, distant. They now became quiet, proud, beautiful, animated, relaxed, involved and able to share and support. When she walked on wearing her outfit, the audience was seeing a woman who had stature, was confident, and held her head high, as did the others. I however was privileged to see more. A metamorphosis both physical and psychological. She had found her own inner strength reinforced by those around her who were willing to accompany her on some of her personal journey.

Resources

I often 'Google' a topic to help me come up with an idea for a project but this can be time-consuming. Below are a few websites I would recommend:

www.arts.ac.uk – volunteering uin the arts, based at LCF, accessed on 16 February 2008.

www.photojojo.com – I've found this site has a few interesting ideas for photographic projects that are emailed to me regularly. Some I am able to work with, others I am not; still, a useful resource, accessed on 16 February 2008.

'4 free' websites – there are more and more local websites across the country that in the current push for recycling are giving people the opportunity to advertise goods that they are willing to give away for free or in exchange. It's a good idea to occasionally check out for lighting, tripods, lenses and other photographic equipment, accessed on 16 February 2008.

www.myjannee.com – this is a really good site for anyone wanting to get to know Adobe Photoshop CS a little better. Full of useful tips and projects at all levels, accssed on 16 February 2008.

http://digitalmedia.jhu.edu/learning – useful for ideas and technical information, accessed on 16 February 2008.

It is always worth getting in touch with local photographic or video clubs. They are usually very welcoming and willing to offer help and advice and even come to the hospice to give a talk or demo to patients and staff.

www.willowfoundation.org.uk/home.shtml – they organise and finance special days for people who are terminally ill and under the age of 40 years, accessed on 16 February 2008.

www.rosettalife.org – Rosetta Life is an organisation of professional artists that enables people with life-threatening illnesses and their families to explore experiences of significance through video, photography, drama, music, poetry, dance, fiction and other digital art forms, accessed on 16 February 2008.

Appendix

The volunteers in 'Something so Strong':

Caterina Radvan: Visiting Lecturer in Knitwear, Brighton University, 1994–6; Textile Artist in Residence, South East Arts, Uckfield, 1995. Awards: Winner, Marks & Spencer Children's wear Competition, 1993.

Peter Cox: Senior Lecturer at LCF, specialist in tailoring; has worked with many high profile designers such as Stella McCartney.

Natalie Hren: fashion graduate from America now studying textile design for a year at Chelsea Art College.

Daniella Rajdova: studying at Chelsea Art College.

Joining us later on in the project were:

Manjinder: machinist, just graduated from LCF.

Martyn Rose: photographer; website: www.martynrose.co.uk.

10 Art Therapy

Samantha Dobbs

Working as an arts therapist

I joined the hospice arts team as part of my two-year art psychotherapy Master's degree and a permanent position followed my training placement. Art therapy posts are few, so I am delighted to be able to continue as part of the team and offer this service to a range of clients in palliative care. I work one day a week in the day unit as part of the Creative Living Centre, on the wards and in the community.

Art therapy is part of a range of creative arts opportunities used in healthcare since the 1940s. However, making marks and images is a communication activity used since ancient times, an example being cave drawings (Case and Dalley 1992). There is an assumption that in some way creating art or images is good for us. Image-making can tap into an inner reality of the person. Faced with an incurable illness, the client has many challenges and difficulties and art therapy can facilitate communication and expression of these in non-verbal and verbal forms. Making images can bring about personal change in attitudes and feelings. Literature supporting the use of arts therapies in palliative care has been growing since the 1980s (Pratt and Wood 1998).

Art therapists usually have an arts or psychology background or both and hold a professional qualification that is governed and regulated by the Health Professions Council (www.hpc-uk.org). This means we adhere to set guidelines and codes of practice and ethics. To ensure the clients receive the best possible care, we have regular clinical supervision with other art psychotherapists to share clients' work and open up our thinking. I come from an art and nursing background. My nursing history and practice have been invaluable in helping me to engage and work with this client group: I am familiar with the dying body, deteriorating self-image and odours that can accompany incurable illness. My working history has helped me to understand the difficulties of working with the medical model and increasing my flexibility. I am familiar with working in a professional team, and often we provide support to each other, particularly the other arts therapists and art team.

Art therapy in palliative care

Art therapy is a form of therapy using art materials that enable clients to explore emotional and psychological issues. The therapy is not directed by the therapist; rather, clients lead the way. Clients in the palliative care setting often express powerful, difficult emotions concerning their illness, treatment, mortality and life too. I often work with high levels of distress. The ethos of the hospice is 'living' with 'dying', and art therapy can help to address some of the psychological trauma of the realities of living with a terminal illness. Sometimes words cannot be found to explain thoughts and feelings and so image making with support from me can enable communication. We create a reflective space for the clients. The eminent psychoanalyst John Bowlby, advocated that a therapist's 'sensitive responsiveness' (Marrone 1998, p.42) was essential for the cooperation of the client, meaning that the therapist was responsive, empathetic and noticed 'timely signals' (Marrone 1998, p.147). I try to work with sensitive responsiveness to help my clients engage in the process.

Sometimes clients fear that you will be able to see or read things in their images. This is not the case. Art therapists do not interpret the image or artefact. The meaning comes from the client and is never fixed or static, but changeable and can mean many things at once. This is something that can be worked on together. Another fear or myth is that you have to have artistic experience to benefit from this therapy. This is not true. You do not need to be good at art or have any experience of image making to benefit from this psychological support. The focus is on image or artefact making, alongside the process and the relationship with the therapist. This is sometimes referred to as the 'triangular relationship' (Schaverien 1998).

The relationship with the therapist can be a key factor in the therapy. I can explore with the client what is going on in the relationship with us in the room, and with the art or image made. I try to keep the focus on the here and now, what is happening in the present. This can facilitate emotional change and healing. I use myself as a tool in the therapy. Feelings that might emerge for me could be coming up within and be reflected from the client. If the client is able to engage with the therapy at this unconscious level, we may talk about these feelings. This is similar to something called 'resonance'. It means that the therapist can pick up on the feelings from the client in an unconscious way through such subtleties as body language. By looking at the process, I am looking at behaviour and words and image that can inform me about the nature of our relationship and interaction. It is helpful to take a symbolic step back and think: 'What is going on here?'

The relationship with me and the image can enable some conflict to surface and, I hope, to achieve resolution during the sessions. Art therapists are 'aware of the importance of relationships; they are also concerned with what kind of boundaries make the work safe' (Learmonth and Huckvale 2002, p.3). There is a need to 'protect non judgmental creative spaces' (Learmonth and Huckvale 2002, p.3). I try to minimise our interruptions when we work together.

The image is unique and personal. Often it is linked to the person's self-esteem and identity. Art therapy is a space where a new potential identity can be explored with the space and materials. There is a change to sense of self when faced with incurable illness. Image making is another form of communicating; I would say that making the image is like using another language. Making and creating images and artefacts can be like having a conversation or telling a story, the image speaks. The image can be the container for feelings and the image can then be left behind with the therapist.

I discuss with clients what is to be done with the images when the therapy has finished, as part of contract-making at the beginning of the therapy. Usually the therapist holds on to the images until the end of the therapy. The client then has the choice to leave the images with the therapist or to give the images to family or friends. It can be important for the client to leave something behind for family or friends.

Art therapists are psychologically informed. The theory behind the therapy is from psychoanalytic studies, psychotherapy and attachment. Case and Dalley (1992, p.5) state: 'The orientation of the art therapist might be informed by the ideas of Freud, Klein or Jung or more recently, the post-Freudians or such eminent writers as Donald Winnicott, Marion Milner and so on.' I also read the work of the psychotherapist Irvine Yalom. Theory is used to provide some understanding of human behaviour in the inside world and the outside world. Metaphor, symbol and story-telling can inform our practice too. Story-telling can be important and is incorporated into the therapy. One client made up a story about the image she drew in the previous session:

> Once upon a time there was an old balloon seller called Mr Frogmore. An Edwardian lady would buy his balloons for all the children in the park. She would turn up on a Friday morning in her finest bonnet…and the children really loved her because she always bought every one of them a balloon – she never left one of them out.

This is part of the story that reflected her kind and giving nature and her ability to turn sad feelings into happy ones.

Often, clients make symbolic images, holding many meanings. A symbol is a representation of an idea, feeling or thing. A Jungian approach looks at the use of symbols in creativity and therapy and a search for their meaning can heal the 'psyche', soul, spirit (Case and Dalley 1992, p.89). An example of a symbol could be a tree, which can mean literally a tree, or it represents the self, or refers to living organic matter, nature or life (see Connell 1994 for further thoughts on trees). Sometimes clients use metaphors when thinking about their image.

One lady described her image of a winter tree as being like death; using this metaphor enabled her to express herself.

Art therapy practice

The three main settings for my art therapy work are in an art therapy group, or, for individual art therapy, by the bedside or in the designated room. With art therapy, the focus is on the feelings that are aroused when making whatever form of art the client chooses. I follow the art therapy convention discussed above that the image is confidential unless the client wishes the work to be exhibited or shared with others. In comparison, other artists in the arts team focus on the art product and may offer a form of teaching. Both art and art therapy offer support but the therapist thinks about the psychodynamics of the relationship and the unconscious process.

When working at the bedside, I visit clients in the hospice with my art trolley. I can offer the client paint, acrylic paint, watercolours, pastels, crayons, felt tip pens, pencils, clay, plasticine, collage material, glue, scissors, assorted paper and card, the list goes on. I aim to see the client for the usual 50-minute therapeutic hour, following psychoanalytic practice, but this is a guide only. Some clients are too sick to tolerate a full 50 minutes, so we sometimes spend less time together. The session is client-led in both time and content.

I also offer art therapy to people in the community, taking a small mobile art therapy box of supplies to nursing homes. This is similar to seeing someone in the hospice wards: usually they are in a self-contained room that is like a mini-home for them; in the case of those in the hospice this is temporary, in that of those in nursing homes, more permanent. I clear a space to work in before beginning, and try to work as cleanly as possible at the bedside. Clients can be inhibited by fear of spoiling the bedding. I keep the images stored with me until the end of the therapy as usual in art therapy practice.

Art therapy in a group setting involves an invitation to clients from the wards to come to the group that I hold in the day unit for an hour and a half every week. I understand that this amount of time is too much for some inpatient clients, and a tea break halfway gives group members the option to leave at this point. In palliative care, you have to be flexible because illness and treatments may make people tired. It is about finding a way of working that feels safe enough for you and your clients. The establishment of start and end times, and sticking to them, creates a feeling of safety. Running over time may suggest to the clients that the therapy is not contained. To be contained is to be held and safe. The group is also open to carers and families who may wish to join in and explore some of the feelings, relationships and memories that come up through image making. The nature of groupwork is inspiring as the clients can help each other along with image making and themes that can come up. They can get a sense of belonging in groupwork and feel that 'I'm not the only one'. Clients usually offer support to one another when they talk about their circumstances.

The model of groupwork I am developing is based on the open art studio model. The focus is on creating images, an empathetic environment and respect for each other and each other's image making, not the unconscious processes, although I will make links with the image making in the group. The group dynamic is different every time.

In introducing myself, I say who I am and I give a brief overview of what art therapy can be, such as 'a time and space for you to express yourself using the art materials however you chose'. I have a leaflet at the hospice that gives a few more details and providing the clients can read I leave an information leaflet with them when we first meet before we have an assessment session. This assessment session is a time for me to gain a little insight into the client's world; some behaviour patterns may start to emerge. I ask a series of questions that give me what I need before we start a therapy process. I put up 'Please Do Not Disturb' signs to try and ensure that it is an uninterrupted space. Keeping the space safe from interruptions is an important element in art therapy. Eventually the client can trust that the space is protected and this can be supportive and holding.

As with individual sessions, whatever is made in the group is confidential and the therapy is private. Clients may choose what to do with the images made at the end of the sessions or in the event of their death. Some wish me to keep their work, others pass the work onto their family, and one wished her art to be displayed at her wake. I explain at the beginning that I have a supervisor with whom I share my work. I also explain that I will write in their patients' notes after a session that I have seen them; I share a brief overview of the session with the multidisciplinary team in this way. So it is not always completely confidential, but I honour the clients' wishes whatever happens.

It can feel intimidating and threatening to be in a room with a new person who comes with a selection of art materials and paper. I have heard many times: 'I've not made art since school'; on further engagement, I have discovered that usually these clients didn't have a good experience of art at school. This can result in some people finding it hard to start with the image making, since they are looking for some direction. I try gently to encourage the client to choose a material to work with, and to see where it goes. One woman was nervous about starting and a bit sceptical, but, after choosing oil pastels and a small piece of paper, she was delighted to discover that she could make sensitive images which I thought beautiful. She liked the result and gained a sense of purpose from the therapy. On other occasions when it is hard to begin, I interact with the client by getting us both to make a mark on a page with a pen, felt-tip marker or pencil; in this way we begin to engage. This method was first used by Winnicott (1971) when he was trying to engage his young clients with art materials; he called it the 'squiggle game'. With adults who are first embarking on art therapy, I do not use the terms 'game' or 'play' since often they complain it feels a bit silly when they are unsure what to do, what to expect or what to produce. I ask if they would like to start with choosing a colour and then make a mark, I will follow that mark with my own and then we can see what happens.

Responses

Providing art therapy in palliative care can be profoundly moving as the client struggles to come to terms with the initial diagnosis or the diagnosis of being in a terminal phase of their illness. It can be helpful to be aware of Kübler-Ross's (1970) stages of death and dying: grief, anger, acceptance, shock, depression, bargaining and denial. Clients may go through these stages at any time, and in no particular order. The issue of control is often present and powerful. In palliative care or after a particularly lengthy period of medical treatment, clients often feel that they have no control over their illness, their treatment, the progress and life in general. They may also have lack of control over their bodily functions, which contributes to the powerlessness (Waller and Sibbett 2005). They seem to have many things done to them. This is discussed by other art therapy authors (Pratt and Wood 1998; Waller and Sibbett 2005). The clients are in a medical model of care where the focus can be on the disease rather than what else is going on for them emotionally and psychologically. Art therapy provides the opportunity to have some control. They control the materials they use, they can choose the depths to which they go with the image making and the story-telling and sometimes the length of the sessions. This can provide the opportunity for the client to take back some power and control through their active participation in sessions.

I find that art and image making is therapeutic in its own right and this is why I became an art therapist. I use image making myself to process and open up emotions and thoughts. It is fascinating for me and I find my clients are interested and fascinated too. There is something about the nature of creating that can take you onto another level of thinking, existing and philosophising. One client found some startling revelations about her personal space and relationship after contemplating her abstract painting. She made an image using bold coloured acrylics. This elicited a response concerning her body, we were able to talk about how separated she felt from her own body, and the internal bruising she felt, expressed by a thick purple line. During this session, she discovered that she had been shying away from physical contact with her partner, because she felt so vulnerable and bruised. Through the image, she was able to see that she had been pushing him away, when in fact she needed intimacy. It was a real 'eye-opener' she said.

Image making is like a conduit, and it can also be a container for emotions, a symbolic pot where you can put your emotions, stories and thoughts. The pot may be shaken up and then we see what happens. One client literally made a pot in her final session, and proceeded to make four bits of 'shit' to put in her pot, which was then a potty (a toddler's portable toilet) for her as a child; her potty contained the anger she felt for a shit childhood. Each piece of shit was for a family member and in sharing her anger she was able to acknowledge it, feel it and then bring it in to the present and relate it to how angry she felt that she was dying, dying was shit and she was angry about it. After this release she was able to move onto a more peaceful image.

Art therapy is client-led. I try to follow the client in the therapy and to see them with new eyes each time, or have a 'beginner's mind' (McNiff 1992). I work with an active mind and I try and pay full attention to the client. It is like being in the client's world but not a part of it. I aim to be significantly removed to be of value to the client. I consider as I work the philosophy of the psychotherapist Yalom, who holds his patients with 'unconditional positive regard', a term from Rogers's (2003) person-centred humanistic model of therapy. Yalom is an existential psychotherapist, which means he works with the issues that concern us all about our existence such as 'Death, Isolation, the Meaning of life, and Freedom' (see Yalom website). This form of therapy looks also at the inner world, conflict and trauma plus these 'givens'. Existential psychotherapy assumes that unconscious forces influence conscious functions (see Yalom website). Art therapy looks at unconscious processes. I try not to approach the therapy with an agenda of my own as this can leave you 'narcissistically wounded' as a therapist, which means you leave yourself open to pain and self-criticism (Casement 2002).

People who are wondering about therapy with terminal or progressive illness sometimes ask: 'What is the point?' 'In palliative care, what can you hope to achieve?' I think that the release and witnessing of difficult emotions often provides comfort to clients. Art therapy is used to decrease pain and in some cases can help the inevitable ending. Clients who are suffering emotionally can have a lower threshold to physical pain and so art therapy has an important role on a physical level (Thomas 1995). If some of the feelings and emotions that clients find uncomfortable can be left behind, they may be able to think and feel differently. Image making and art can be a search for meaning that is often important at the end of life. It can be a space to explore their identity that has been changing though the nature of suffering disease, illness and treatment.

It is a privilege to witness the journey, the pain, the realisations, the changes that clients may make. The therapy together can be short term or for a longer journey. Clients who have had one session have plunged right in to the deep and meaningful questions and struggles they are having. Perhaps this is because they have a different notion about time, since issues may arise quickly when you know you are dying and your time is limited (Connell 1992; Pratt and Wood 1998; Thomas 1995; Waller and Sibbett 2005). Clients can find release in expressing feelings, and having them shared and witnessed can be important. Sometimes, a little of their pain is left behind with me in the image.

I will now present two case studies: names are changed, no specific age or diagnosis is offered to provide some confidentiality and permission has been given.

Case study: Anne

Anne was a woman in her early fifties. She was diagnosed with a cancerous tumour in the summer months; this quickly progressed to multiple tumours in the autumn. I saw her for three very powerful, moving sessions. The issue of loss was in the forefront of these sessions. She compared the years of her life to the seasons and she felt that as a 50-year-old she should be enjoying the autumn season of her life and early retirement. Cancer made her feel as though she had lost a whole 'season' of her life. For her it was the winter, she was coming to the end of her life, and it should have been her autumn season. She was able to symbolise this in an image of a tree. She showed me on paper with poster paints how she felt about winter and her potential death. She then reflected how she felt; she felt sad and lonely and the image was sad and lonely. Dying can be lonely and isolating even when you're surrounded by loved ones. It is a very individual experience and everyone's death is different for them.

We started the following session as we had before. Anne wondered what she could do today and was keen to experiment with different materials. She had been thinking about what she could do in the session and as she had used paints in the last session, was enthusiastic to experiment with new material. She created an image with oil pastels and talked about how much hope she had for the future. She really wanted to go home and climb the stairs. Her image showed her in different colours and stages moving up a staircase. I felt unsure whether she was climbing her staircase at home or whether this was a staircase to another dimension beyond living. I reflected this back to her; we were able to explore both possibilities. She recognised herself on each step and how she was struggling to cope with the difficulties of the treatment and the discharge plans. She could also see how when she got to the top of the stairs she was at the edge of the page, and so the future felt beyond the image.

The image following this was made with paint and contained her broken liver and secondary cancer spread. The decline of her health was her first interpretation. This was a bright painted image, though, and later, when contemplating the finished piece, she said if it were her cancer then she would have used darker paint colours and not bright ones. The shapes were then her body parts but the colours felt wrong. She then moved onto another interpretation of her image. This image for her then meant her career path. The spots were her projects and the lines were her work in decline. We contemplated this together and decided that it could mean both things.

As I mentioned earlier, the clients seem to go through a range of emotions about impending death. In her final session, Anne pounded the clay with a nervous laugh which didn't feel funny at all; I thought she was covering up anger with laughter. She was able to share this with me and later said she was expressing her anger. The clay took on a form of a pot of shit, and this was how she felt about where she was. She was dying and it was shit! She was angry.

The image following this was more serene and calm. She formed a shell circle on a midnight blue page and talked of how protected she felt by a circle of people around her. She said that I was there too, in the circle. On that day I was wearing a shell necklace and she commented on this. She also shared a dream that she had in the week where she had been in bed surrounded by a circle of people helping her. She was the pearl in the middle and felt protected and held by the circles. This image was the final one made and for me felt like an ancient meeting place or stone circle where you celebrate life and death. It felt like it was her saying goodbye, it was her midnight blue or twilight hours and, indeed, she died shortly after. I felt her choice of midnight blue was very powerful and the circles emotionally moving.

Anne was able to express many emotions through her image making and told me that, although exhausted after our sessions, she always felt better and comforted. She said the therapy helped her to explore feelings around death and dying, going home, physical contact and the vulnerability of being weak and bedbound. She used image making to release difficult emotions.

Case study: Betty

Betty was in her early sixties and completely debilitated by multiple sclerosis; she was bedbound, dependent on others for almost every need. She had limited mobility in her arms and no strength in her legs. Pain in her back and buttocks prevented her from transferring from her bed into a chair. After our initial meeting, I asked her how many sessions she would like to have with me. She decided to have eight sessions in total and I was pleased since I felt she needed to have this control; it offered some balance to the feeling that she had lost control of her physical functions.

The issue of control is very relevant when working with clients who have cancer or other incurable, deteriorating conditions. She had no control over her body, her bodily functions, her treatment or her daily routine. Waller argues that 'being in control maybe important as the person is losing control of their bodily functions' (2002, p.2). She controlled our length of sessions and end date. She had arms that would jerk out of control, and sometimes this made it difficult for her to use the art materials. I was able to see and feel her frustrations and the torture she suffered 'lying in this bloody bed'.

For one session, we tried another way of working and I offered her the use of my body to make the image. I offered to draw for her under her direction. She still chose the colours, the paper size, what image to put where and how large to draw. She directed my hands. It was the first time I had done this and it felt strange, but it felt particularly useful on the day as she was struggling more than usual to hold the pencils. She seemed to like the result and was relieved not to be juddering so uncontrollably that it became distressing for her. We only worked this way once, because every other session she made her own marks, eventually. It was important to witness and share this struggle; it was part of her showing me how awful it was to have this 'bloody MS'.

In one session, she reminisced about childhood events and memories. Seeing and touching the pencils had stirred up some old stories because when she was a child she really wanted a similar set of pencils but her family were too poor to afford them. One image included here was of an elephant. She liked elephants and shared with me that she was always drawing them as a child; she loved to draw them. I wondered whether the qualities of elephant that she so loved were qualities within her. They were 'loyal and strong'. Betty did not know. She thought that she was loyal but did not seem to be able to think about being strong or not. I wondered whether she felt envy about the strength of the elephant, this elephant strength had wasted away from her by this cruel disease. She felt dissatisfied with this elephant. Its back legs were too fat she said. I said I thought it was beautiful and that it had a gentle quality about it. She laughed; she could not see beyond her own criticisms of the image. She was not able to draw it right.

On our last session, we looked at the work we had made together, and as she looked at me she said 'Yes look, the poor old thing, old and grey and too thin'. And I thought that she really meant her. I had real empathy for her and a sadness about her wasting away and dependency.

Looking back over the images made together was useful. It can be used to look at the journey of the therapy and it can also be used as a session to rethink the images and process new information and old. With Betty, I asked her at the beginning of the sessions whether she wanted to look at last week's image. There was a question about 'cognitive impairment' that she was reported to have. I only came across this once when in one session she was disorientated to time and place and thought I was someone else. Apart from that, I found her cognitively aware, maybe too aware in fact of her physical limitations and control of her life. 'Bloody MS', she would say. 'Bloody MS.' The nurses reported she seemed calmer after our sessions together.

Conclusion

To summarise, I offer clients a safe time and space where they can explore thoughts, feelings and emotions that come up through making images. My focus is on the image made and the sessions are client-led in content and reflective where possible. I offer psychological support on a one-to-one basis or in a group setting. I enjoy my work and it can feel good for both of us when the client can use the therapy to change some of their circumstances and thinking about their situation. I enjoy image making and usually try to explore the materials when clients leave me or I leave them. This is part of my professional and personal processing after sessions. I process my feelings about my clients through image making and through psychodynamic supervision with other art psychotherapists. The work is a challenge and I often see people in a high state of distress. Part of my work is to facilitate emotional release and help them to contain this in the image if possible since sometimes people find it hard to articulate feelings verbally. The therapeutic space can be a place to explore a variety of issues, personal boundaries, identity changes and relationships. It is an intense job but can be very satisfying. Being part of the team is important for support. When things get tough we as a staff group turn to each other and others in our field.

I would like to end this chapter with a poem I wrote after one of my clients died. I use creativity to process my feelings about my clients whether this is in the form of an image or a piece of creative writing. The creative outlet related to art therapy is important to the therapist and the client. The therapist has to have open thinking and feelings. Creativity following client sessions can help with the internal self-supervisor and is therefore important. I think this poem expresses the depth of the work we can go to with clients:

> I lit a candle for you today,
> To say goodbye, Good luck on your journey,
> I hope you're smiling and at peace
> Wherever that maybe.
>
> I have pondered over your images,
> I have thought about us together,
> I can say how profoundly moved I am,
> That you have left the world forever.
>
> It was a great honour to witness,
> How you made such deep unconscious art,
> You were brave to experiment and make mess,
> How you poured these from your heart.
>
> I was witness to your emotions,
> It was an amazing and special time,
> I didn't realise how connected we were
> The impact was quite sublime.

Further reading

Case, C. and Dalley, T. (1992) *The Handbook of Art Therapy*. London: Routledge.

This book is a good introduction to the world of art therapy, including chapters on the art therapy room, the therapy in art therapy and developing psychoanalytic understanding.

Farrelly-Hansen, M. (2001) *Spirituality and Art Therapy: Living the Connection*. London: Jessica Kingsley Publishers.

This is an edited collection whose chapters show different ways of thinking about art therapy and healing in the therapeutic approach. The book looks at using nature, transpersonal psychology, and Jewish, Celtic and Shamanistic perspectives. All very interesting for opening up your thinking.

Waller, D. and Sibbett, C. (eds) (2005) *Facing Death: Art Therapy and Cancer Care.* Buckingham: Open University Press.

This is a well-referenced and well-researched book about cancer and looks in depth at transference and counter-transference issues. I recommend reading it because they are hugely influential aspects of therapy that I have not included in this chapter.

Websites

www.baat.org – British Association of Art Therapists, accessed on 16 February 2008.

www.creativeresponse.org.uk – Creative Response is a special site for palliative care, Aids, cancer and loss, accessed on 16 February 2008.

www.hpc-uk.org – website of the Health Professions Council which regulates the arts therapies, accessed on 16 February 2008.

www.yalom.com.htm – Yalom website, accessed on 16 February 2008.

11 Community Arts

Virginia Hearth

Applying community arts experience to creative arts in palliative care

In January 2007, St Christopher's Hospice set up a community arts project called 'Arts for Life', made possible with two-year funding from Arts Council England. I am one of the three community artists employed on the project to work with some of the hospice's most vulnerable patients in their own homes, nursing homes and residential homes. Prior to starting this project, I had been working in South Wales for several years as a community artist. I formerly trained as a visual artist and a counsellor and I am currently training in arts psychotherapy. I work part-time for St Christopher's and for the remainder of my time I work as a freelance community artist in South Wales and London; I am in the process of relocating my studio.

Starting out to write this chapter with no prior experience of working in palliative care enables me to apply a rich community arts experience to a new setting. I hope to convey an impression of the work that I do and why it matters in the hope that others find the inspiration to work in a similar way.

St Christopher's Hospice, in more than 40 years' work, has sought to make the arts integral to the care available to patients. It prides itself on quality of care and innovation, and it is this vision that has led to the development of the Creative Living Centre within the hospice and to the 'Arts for Life' project. The hospice aims to include the contribution of creative arts in understanding and responding to patients' needs in a positive, innovative and creative manner. This project sits within the Creative Living Centre, which includes complementary therapists, physiotherapists, hairdressers, gardeners and horticulturists, and the arts team. In addition to the community artists, the arts team consists of two hospice-based artists, two music therapists and an art therapist plus students on placements.

The modern hospice movement was developed through a desire to reduce the isolation that patients and their families can experience in hospitals whose conventions mean that a dying patient is set apart in many dimensions from their family and self. The hospice movement was radical in that it challenged respect for authority, faith in medicine and fear of illness and death, instead embracing death as a final stage of growth and grief as a process of healing. Over the years, palliative care has extended out into the community, however, the arts and complementary therapies have generally been hospice-based. This means that these services have become exclusive to those who are fortunate enough to be able to access the hospice. The 'Arts for Life' project, through developing a community arts approach, sets out to rebalance this inequality and to reduce the isolation patients face in the community as well as in a hospice setting.

Care packages at home are often comprehensive, with several visits per day from healthcare professionals, but this can still be a very lonely time. With great attention being given to the body, the many other facets that make a person whole can feel neglected leading to a sense of disorientation, disassociation and a loss of identity. The person can become 'lost' in their illness, feeling that the illness is permeating not just their physical being but also their whole world. It is a basic human need to be recognised and understood, and this is the foundation upon which positive relationships are formed. When people are nearing death, it is all the more important that they feel understood and recognised in order to feel very much alive and present.

Patients receiving care at home can sometimes feel more vulnerable and less defended against the fears that close proximity to death can bring than people in a hospice. These people do not have the advantages of being part of a group at the day unit, where patients can share their experiences with other members of the group. The 'Arts for Life' project recognises people's needs and responds by enabling them to express themselves creatively, so that they are less likely to suffer from isolation and depression. Feedback from our patients suggests that creativity matters to them.

Through offering a wide range of choice to patients we aim to reinforce a sense of control at a time when people can feel helpless. We do not place a greater or lesser importance on the 'Arts for Life' project as opposed to day unit arts workshops. This recognises the value and diversity of the different options available to patients, and recognises the diverse needs of patients in a flexible approach. We work together to find the most appropriate service for a person, taking into consideration their needs, circumstances and preferences.

Such an approach embraces the arts as an alternative complementary medicine for people who are reaching the end of their life; medicine for the soul. Creativity is not a panacea but provides a means of transport into the imagination, where anything is possible, where even the most difficult issues and emotions can be addressed. The arts can help to demystify death and dying, which can be a source of relief and comfort for patients, their families and the wider community. They can act as a vehicle for expressing the inexpressible courageously and without censorship and can encompass the whole of our being, containing our feelings with dignity and respect.

The arts offer us a way of making sense of the world and help us to define who we are and who we have been: 'Our mind works in pictures, not words, and we grapple to express the inexpressible' (Waller and Sibbet 2005, p.4). Throughout history artists, poets, writers, musicians, playwrights, dancers and puppeteers have used metaphor to mystically reveal wisdom through their creativity. Death has always been an inspiration for artistic imagination: 'No thought exists in me which death has not carved with his chisel' (Michelangelo, quoted in Sheikh 2003, p.472).

Death is of course part of life and cannot be denied, although contemporary western society can be prone to neuroses around this aspect of life. Taboos are riddled with shame, and death and dying are taboo subjects in many cultures, particularly Western society. People's reluctance to discuss death or avoidance of any confrontation with their own mortality or the mortality of others reflects the taboo. The arts can enable us to face our greatest fears and shames, and through coming to terms with death many people can better appreciate the many things they enjoy in life.

The sensitivity and courage of the artist to walk with a patient into their internal landscape is an art in itself. The art of this is instinctual, provided the artist has a well-developed sense of empathy, congruence and unconditional positive regard. These are the core conditions that inform person-centred therapy, developed by Carl Rogers (2005). Later on I explore the subject of training for artists working in healthcare settings, touching on the current debate around arts therapies and arts in health.

Other elements of the 'Arts for Life' project include regular high-profile exhibitions within the catchment communities that the hospice covers, training and conferences on arts in palliative care, an online forum for artists and arts therapists working in palliative care, and community-based arts workshops with a focus on promoting healthier attitudes to death, dying and bereavement. The arts are particularly useful for helping to address the issues of terminal illnesses, death and bereavement through the use of metaphor. For example, projects that we have done in the past have focused on beginnings and endings, journeys and change, and have used metaphors such as butterflies, rivers, dusk and dawn, the seasons and the elements. We work directly on the conception and delivery of projects with partner organisations. Community arts in this context act as a bridging medium between the hospice and the wider community. It is important that hospices challenge the myth that they are the social space of the condemned.

The work of community artists differs from that of arts therapists in that it is not part of a prescribed treatment and is not clinical. Its therapeutic effects come from creativity in general and from a relationship with the artist. Within the Creative Living Centre at St Christopher's, the differentiation between artists and arts therapists is clear. Creative tensions within the field of the arts, including community arts, arts in healthcare settings and arts therapies, are discussed as part of the evolution of our arts team; it is from this dialogue that some of the richest practice can evolve because our intentions are clear and we co-exist harmoniously without the blurring of boundaries or duplication. Within this organisation we have brought a myriad of arts practices and expertise together to form our multi-professional arts team. Time is the major barrier for the cohesion of this team and, whilst a mutual respect exists, co-working in its true sense is yet to occur. When it does, I believe we will model something for the national and international arts community.

Supervision and self-support systems

To ensure the success of any arts practice within a hospice setting, support is necessary from managers, funders and the professionals who work within the field of palliative care. Clinical supervision must be regarded as an essential element for any arts practice within healthcare, particularly if ongoing relationships with patients are a part of the work of the artist. Supervision should not be provided by a colleague or manager but by an independent clinical supervisor so that a process of supportive exploration can be provided. This provides artists with the space and permission for reflection and, without this, artists' interventions are at risk of becoming emotional reactions rather than creative responses.

A question that our nurses ask our patients is 'What helps you to cope?' I feel that this is an important question to ask ourselves whatever our role may be within palliative care services. I encourage the staff that I work with to use the arts to consider their coping systems and what they may need more of to feel supported. Personally, I need to feel a part of a team and to know that people are there to catch me when I fall. I also need to express myself creatively to process the emotional responses that I feel from this work. I paint, write, dance and sculpt to keep myself healthy. A simple journal can be a good way to start people off: just writing down one word at the end of the day may help staff to bracket off the work from their personal lives.

Being part of a team

It is important that artists do not feel isolated within a hospice, particularly as the artist will be working to address isolation for patients. Building recognition by other professionals so that the contribution of artists is valued can lead to a sense of inclusion for the artist. If the artist is working to promote inclusion and self-esteem for patients it is important that they too feel valued by the organisation of which they are a part.

One way to achieve this is to include staff and volunteers in projects. At the hospice, we undertook a mural project 100 feet long. Over 300 people took part including patients and their families and friends, staff ranging from kitchen staff to consultants, volunteers and the wider community. Staff would work during their lunch hour on the project as they felt it was therapeutic and were excited by both the process and the product. The project changed the atmosphere and culture of the hospice as everyone worked together to achieve a shared goal. I also run training sessions to staff teams throughout the hospice to educate them about the work that we do and to let them experience it for themselves. It is only through doing that people gain understanding.

Creative arts in advocacy

I wonder at my motivation for wanting to develop this side of my practice and suspect that it is born from my own frustrations and a desire to empower patients. I would like to use creative arts in advocacy to give voice to those that are strong in spirit but weak in body. I would like to use the arts to help change policies and funding decisions that have a direct impact on the quality of life for people with terminal illness. The arts are powerful and speak to the heart, a language that we all can understand if we take notice.

Case studies

The following case studies illustrate the way in which I work as a community artist in palliative care. Keeping a journal is an important process for planning my work, for supervision and for professional reflection. I provide examples of journal entries to illustrate the emotional impact that this work has upon me and my own creativity.

I shall return to my very first patient and shall refer to her as Emma to protect her anonymity. Emma was referred to me because she was an elderly woman who was socially isolated. Having been a very active and hard-working woman, Emma was housebound due to emphysema. Her oxygen supply meant that it was difficult to leave the house; she struggled with anxiety and panic attacks. I met Emma at home with her husband and she was comfortable in talking about her life and her acceptance of death. She also spoke of her career and her country of origin. We explored ways in which we might work together, although Emma was clear from the start that she did not want to draw or paint. Emma liked the sound of guided imagery relaxation, which I described as a journey into the imagination, helping Emma to paint pictures in her mind. She also wanted to read poems and she told me the names of some of her favourite poets.

The following week I returned to Emma's home with a poetry book, some writing materials (in case Emma was inspired to write her own poem), some visual arts materials (I had a hunch that the guided imagery exercise might provoke a desire to work with visual imagery) and a relaxation technique and guided imagery exercise in mind. For some time, we read poems aloud to each other, many of them being favourites of Emma's and triggering memories. Emma expressed a readiness to try the relaxation technique and guided imagery.

I used a technique that I learnt many years ago and have used many times as a way of helping people to access their imaginations. I started the guided imagery in a meadow, and then journeyed into a forest, all the time helping Emma to connect with her senses through her imagination. The guided imagery ends on a boat on a lake as the sun is setting. I asked Emma to pay particular attention to her feelings and body as she journeyed through her imagination. For Emma, this was very effective and she was quite excited by the things that she had sensed and felt. Emma then asked to see the visual arts materials that I had brought with me, so I showed her the selection of drawing and painting materials. She was drawn to the chalk pastels and some purple sugar paper and was mobilised until the point at which a pastel was in her hand but she didn't have the confidence to make contact with the paper. Emma became stuck, with her trembling hand suspended above the paper, too afraid to go any further. Emma believed that she had never been any good at art and that her teachers had told her this, a story that I have heard many times. This imposed self-concept stays with many people. Regardless of my reassurance, Emma was terrified. At this stage, I was concerned that Emma would be overwhelmed with fear. Having got this far with Emma, I didn't want to turn back. I offered to draw with her, something that is contradictory to my integrative arts psychotherapy training.

And so I made the first marks and Emma followed, and the marks were almost like strokes on the paper, rhythmical and comforting. And gradually, her marks began to take a form. It was a fascinating process, almost as if we were dancing on the page. Emma's marks became more definite and deliberate and took the form of a beautiful flower. Emma's attention then turned to the roots of the flower and the soil, and she used her fingers to blend the earthy colours. She became very focused on the soil and the roots and I withdrew from the page. I am not sure that she noticed this as she continued with deliberateness.

Emma decided that her drawing was completed and showed it to her husband with pride. He was surprised and complimentary, which pleased her. Emma thanked me and said that she had never thought she could do something like that. She died shortly after this.

When I heard that Emma had died, I had an urge to look at her drawing. It felt sacred, and I realised at that point just how important art is. So much of Emma was in her drawing and I saw the beauty of her soul. This experience set a precedent for my work and how I say goodbye to patients and process loss for myself.

Another patient that I worked with was a woman in her forties with cancer whom I shall call Dawn. I had just two meetings with Dawn before she died. Dawn had wanted to use watercolours, as this was the medium that she was most competent with. She actually used chalk pastels, as she wanted to try something new. She knew precisely what she wanted to draw – a window and a mirror. I asked Dawn what the window and the mirror meant for her. She said that she had wanted to paint the window, as it was a window with a view of one of her favourite places. She didn't know why she wanted a mirror in the picture. Towards the end of the session, she said that actually it was a window to the next world, and said goodbye.

Of course, windows and mirrors are two of the oldest and most powerful metaphors recognised within art history, and psychotherapy recognises these as archetypal imagery. Foucault (1986, p.24) suggests that in the mirror 'I discover my absence from the place where I am since I see myself over there' and 'I come back toward myself; I begin again to direct my eyes toward myself and to reconstitute myself there where I am'. I think it helped Dawn to prepare for her death, which happened just a few days after this drawing was made.

Luke (a disguised name) is a man in his early sixties. He collapsed on holiday and has not been able to walk since then. His paralysis is due to cancer. He had been working right up until that point and is now bedbound. The adjustment for Luke has been very difficult and a wait for adaptations to his home makes the adjustment even more difficult as he is now dependent on others for many aspects of daily living.

The first time I saw Luke he could speak of nothing else other than his frustration and despair with his situation. He did not see how creativity could possibly help him. The power of his communication of anger and frustration with weaknesses in care services stimulated my empathy with his predicament and this made me wonder how helpful I could be for Luke. However, he talked a little about his relationship with his grandmother and how important that was when he was a child. He spoke about the first time he came to Britain and first saw snow. I offered to help Luke to record these stories in a creative way, possibly through film or creative writing but he didn't want to do this. He asked what else we could do together and so I went through different art forms that might be available to him. When I mentioned painting, he responded positively, and so I rearranged another appointment to return with some paints.

On returning to the hospice, I spoke to colleagues about his situation and we discussed the reality for a great many patients that services cannot respond to the needs that they feel. This is difficult for me, and all of us, to accept and challenge. I am still wondering about the scope for using the arts as a tool for raising awareness about needs for care services. Later on I discuss project ideas that I plan to realise.

I returned the following week with watercolours. Luke was disappointed to realise that he had a blank piece of paper to work with and felt that this was too much of a challenge for him. I encouraged him to just see what would emerge and reassured him. I gave him a demonstration of what was possible with the medium and how to obtain different results. He experimented a little but then wanted to move on to actually creating something. He played around with shape and colour, asking for advice along the way about colours. Luke was uncertain and I felt as if my role was metaphorically to hold his hand. We spent almost two hours together, and during this time I noticed that the walls in Luke's bedroom were bare.

On finishing his painting Luke was pleased with his achievement and was surprised at how quickly the time had passed. Also, he appeared surprised at how long he had been able to sit upright in bed and not feel pain. I think it was these two factors that helped Luke to realise the value of this experience and so he asked if I would come the following week. He specifically asked for more preparation from me, in drawing something out so that he had something to work with. I asked him what he would like me to draw and he spontaneously announced 'a lion'. I gave him the option of either using watercolours again or another medium. Luke was keen to try something new and so I thought acrylic paints would provide him with a very different experience. I also commented on the lack of anything visual on the walls and that perhaps some of his paintings could go on the walls. He laughed and said that it would depend on what they looked like. I made this observation because I empathised with him and felt that I would need something visually stimulating around me to look at should I find myself bedbound. Over time I have come to realise that Luke intends to walk again and that it is his intention for the spare bedroom that he now resides in to be a vacant room once again.

Several sessions were spent on his 'brave lion' acrylic painting, which I framed. I also laminated several colour and black and white copies to give to friends and family. Members of his family were very impressed as he gave away the copies. The painting is situated in the living room. I hope that his carers and other healthcare professionals see this painting, as they may see Luke in a different way, for his brave lion painting says much about Luke himself: he is a proud, strong and brave man.

Following this, Luke was keen to do another painting. He wanted a painting of birds and then a painting of a horse. These are both silk paintings, which has been Luke's preferred medium so far. I have also done a portrait of Luke, which led to a discussion on the difference of the colour of our skin. We told each other that we accepted each other despite our differences and Luke shook my hand and said, 'I am glad you are here, Gini. You brighten up my life.' I told Luke that I felt honoured to know him.

Responses

I enjoy working with Luke. He is courageous in his art as well as in his attitude to life. In fact, I enjoy working with every person that I am referred. I feel honoured to be able to work so intimately with people, often at their bedside in their own homes and processing many difficult emotions about life and its coming to an end. I also have the privilege of spending time with families, helping family members to see a new aspect to their loved ones. The families benefit from having a legacy in the form of their beloved's art work, and the patients have the joy of being able to create things that they know will live beyond themselves and will be treasures to family and friends. From the feedback that I have received from the nursing teams with whom I work, I help them to gain greater depth in their understanding of patients. Often the arts will enable people to disclose information that can help us to gain a better understanding of the patient and therefore meet their needs more accurately.

Examples of journal entries

This is an excerpt from my journal. I use my journal to process and reflect, to log ideas, to express myself through creativity and as a form of diary.

15 January

Today was my first day in my new job as a community artist at St Christopher's Hospice. I was late because I got lost and found myself in Croydon trapped on a one-way system. It took me over two hours to get there, which left me feeling frustrated and distressed. It took me almost just as long to get home. It worries me that I am going to be lost a lot of the time as the job involves travelling around London. It's also very easy to get lost in the hospice itself because it's such a complicated building.

My first impressions were just how calm, caring and friendly it is at the hospice. The grounds are so beautiful and peaceful and everyone has time for you. I was put at ease about being late, and it was something that I could laugh about by the end of the day.

I went out on a home visit with Elaine who is a complementary therapist. We went to see a lady with MND – motor neurone disease. I didn't know much about this disease until today and I realise just how awful it is. The lady that we went to see had lost all movement apart from the ability to blink. Her husband and daughter seemed very distressed. Elaine asked me how I might work with a patient like this, and the only thing I could think of at the time was perhaps to work with her and the family. I could work with someone like her if only to play music, sing, read poems or stories. I realise now just how creative this job is going to be; I will have to be creative to find ways in which I can engage people who are very limited in what they can do physically.

When I arrived home I asked my partner if I smelled of death. He was shocked by this and so was I. I obviously felt that there was something of the hospice left with me and so I had a shower. I wonder whether it is normal to feel this way or is it something to be ashamed of. I don't know, but it's the truth.

I feel so lucky to have this job. I just know it's going to be a great job.

20 February 2007

One month has passed and I am already in full flow, doing a project with a school and a patient caseload. The job has made me think about my own mortality far more than I had anticipated. It has also changed the way I think about art. I realise the value of art, particularly in that it lives beyond the lives of ourselves and holds so much of who we are. It has also changed the way I think about life, and how I live my own life. I imagine there will be more change ahead.

6 July 2007

Sometimes dying is beautiful and sometimes dying is ugly. I hope I do something to help make death a better experience for people and their families. I hope not to die a horrible death.

9 July 2007

Coming up to six months of me being in the job. Everyone in the arts team works part-time and so it is difficult for us to see each other. It would be impossible to meet once a week and so we have long periods of time where we don't meet up. I feel that its important and special for me to feel part of a close team so that I don't feel isolated and alone with what I carry.

I have been a part of the final days of the lives of loved ones and this has been a very different experience to the experience I have now as an artist working with the dying. I can't quite put it into words: it goes beyond words. I feel as if I am in that strange place between life and death where time and space distort, and some moments feel eternal. What I find most difficult is entering back into the world where time and space seem normal, but somehow absurd, as if humanity is lacking what it is to be human. I have read about this space, referred to as liminal space or 'heteretopia'. It is a place of ambiguity, neither here nor there, betwixt and between. I imagine that this is what patients experience, and I experience it too, perhaps as a parallel process. It fascinates me, and my awareness of it is healthy for it will ensure that I remain grounded and solid.

Comment in journal entries

Reading over these diary entries, I realise just how much the job affects my own life, in a positive way I believe. I am more reflective about my own life and I am grateful for the quality of life and good health that I have:

To be near someone who is dying almost inevitably causes us at some point to reflect on our own mortality, and this 'empathy' can occasionally alarm us; our feelings about the dying and death fluctuate between ourselves and the dying person. (Waller and Sibbet 2005, p.4)

Conclusion

I benefit from having had training in counselling skills and arts therapies, although this is not essential. What this training has done for me is develop my self-awareness and understanding of the significance of the arts. It has also given me the confidence to be with another and to be with feelings, both of which are necessary skills for this job. It is of course essential to have skills in the arts, and to understand what art means for yourself.

I feel that any experience of either working in palliative care or caring for a relative or friend would benefit someone working in this position. Certainly, my own experience of caring for a relative has helped me to understand the pressures that families can face, and what it is to be with someone as they are dying.

The qualities that make up Rogers's (2003) core conditions for person-centred work, discussed above, are also important. These qualities are important and should not be underestimated, because they enable a therapeutic relationship to develop, and it is this that is as important for patients as the making of the arts.

And something that becomes more apparent for me is the importance of being an artist. I feel that it is important to be a practising artist, for it is through the arts that the challenging parts of the work can be processed, and integrity and congruence can be retained. Keeping a private journal of images and text is useful, and ensuring that your own creativity is witnessed is also important as it is for patients. Through the arts we can be seen, and this is affirming and empowering. It is important that, in being an artist working in palliative care, the artist within is not ignored.

Further reading

Artlink (2005) *Extraordinary Everyday: Further Explorations in Collaborative Art in Health Care.* Edinburgh: Artlink.

Gill, S. and Fox, J. (2004) *The Dead Good Funerals Book.* Carlisle: Engineers of the Imagination.

Knight, K. and Schwarzman, M. (2005) *Beginners Guide to Community-Based Arts.* Oakland CA: New Village Press.

Pratt, A. and Thomas, G. (2002) *Guidelines for Arts Therapists and the Arts in Palliative Care Settings.* London: Hospice Information.

Senior, P. and Croall, J. (1993) *Helping to Heal: Arts in Health Care.* London: Calouste Gulbenkian Foundation.

Walker-Kuhne, D. (2005) *Invitation to the Party: Building Bridges to the Arts, Culture and Community.* New York: Theatre Communications Group.

Websites

http://forums.stchristophers.org.uk – the website of the hospice arts forum hosted by St Christopher's Hospice for everyone working in the creative arts in palliative care, accessed on 16 February 2008.

www.hi-arts.co.uk/arts_health.htm – imaginative website from Highlands and Islands Arts, with a good section on arts and health, accessed on 16 February 2008.

www.communityarts.net – the website of the Community Arts Network., accessed on 16 February 2008.

www.welfare-state.org – the archive website of this now closed radical arts organisation, accessed on 16 February 2008.

www.artscouncil.org.uk – the website of Arts Council England, gives access to other Arts Council websites, accessed on 16 February 2008.

www.britishcouncil.org/arts – arts website of the British Council, which represents the UK on arts and cultural matters across the UK, accessed on 16 February 2008.

www.sanctuaryweb.com – website of an American organisation concerned with survival after traumatic experience; offers a range of products, services and training, accessed on 16 February 2008.

12 Beginning to Work as a Community Artist in Palliative Care

Mick Sands

Being new as an artist to palliative care

I am new to palliative care, taking up a part-time post as a community artist at St Christopher's Hospice, fitting in with my work as a musician and composer in a number of different worlds. In professional theatre, I have written or adapted music for productions of classical plays for nearly 20 years. In the world of ethnic and traditional folk music, I am a singer and flute-player with a particular interest in singing styles. For 30 years, I have worked with adults with learning disabilities using drama and music.

As a community artist I have a broad arts brief, to 'develop and maintain a flexible community arts service for patients and carers as part of a new "Arts for Life"' project. Of course, I will do this as a member of a team with a variety of areas of expertise but I am interested in the description 'flexible...arts service'. It implies lots of things: that it is a service that is led by the needs of its users, principally, but I am struck by the challenge to me as an artist to be flexible. I think I am being challenged to have a flexibility of attitude and response to the world of metaphor and the human imagination. Our arts team brief is to visit patients who are living with their illness at home or in nursing homes, and to make contact with community groups to raise awareness about the work of St Christopher's helping to break down taboos around death and dying in our society.

I begin this work with many questions. I'm not even sure if they are the right ones. What will the appropriate response be to the needs of patients? Will I be accepted as part of a multi-professional team that includes doctors, nurses, social workers, physiotherapists? How can I collaborate with my fellow visual artists and also art and music therapists working at the hospice? Will we speak the same language? What difference can I make to people facing the ending of their life? What right do I have to be involved? What is my purpose as an artist in palliative care?

On my side is the instinct that informs my professional work as an artist; singing and playing, creating songs and writing music by myself and with others is one of the ways I express and value myself as a human being. I extend myself and become more myself. I respond to my experience of the world. There is a creative instinct in every human being and I think my role is to honour and witness that quality in each of the people I work with. My question about what right I have to be involved is the wrong question because it leads to questions about my own worthiness; that is not the issue. The wrong question, however, does help. Involvement is not a right but a privilege and is by invitation. My first step therefore is 'to put myself at the disposal' of the patient or carer and see what happens.

I was made warmly welcome at my first home care team meeting and listened carefully as nurse and social worker members of the team introduced patients and questions about how best they might be supported. I became aware that I was gradually being overwhelmed by the complexity and variety of pain that was being talked about, that patients' management of the pain of their illness was complicated by their personal histories, family division, estrangement, the needs of children, partners and parents, their physical home circumstances. I was at a loss. I had difficulty steadying myself to take in what was being said. Then I became aware of a bowl of fresh flowers, which had been placed in the centre of the group. Their delicate, transient beauty held my gaze and it became more possible to hear about the impossible burdens people carry. The placing of flowers at the centre of such a meeting reminded me that there is joy and beauty in life, somewhere, as well as pain. I needed it and held onto the image. Our human life is at the same time delicate, vulnerable, suffering and also resilient and enduring.

Becoming possible

Dynamic creative visions are all very well and necessary but my first encounters have introduced me to the importance of patience and persistence in making and keeping contact with people who are referred to me. There are many obstacles in the course of a week that make contact difficult. The part-time nature of my work restricts my availability. Also, the life of an ill person sometimes means that a trip to the doctors or for treatment, the intervention of daily carers, the pain and the depression associated with the illness can be obstacles to meeting. These can be overcome and when a relationship is established and one becomes part of that person's visiting community then something becomes possible.

What exactly becomes possible? I have often worked as a performer and entertainer. Taking ill people's minds off their worries, discomfort and pain is certainly a good thing. But clearly my role is something more than that. It is more about artistic empowerment and helping someone access the medium for themselves, facilitating their own creativity so that we can mutually explore and share our aliveness.

There are of course obstacles to accessing a particular artistic medium. Music, for instance, in our culture is often regarded as a specialist subject, best left to the experts or confined to what can be played on CD, mp3 or mini-disk players. Many people would view an opportunity to make music as more of an ordeal, vulnerable-making, and be very critical of their 'performance' and their level of skill. I imagine the same might be true of other kinds of art. Perhaps some adults consign such aspects of the world of the imagination to childhood. It's important, therefore, to approach music making carefully in a spirit of playfulness and matter-of-factness. The nature of the instruments is important; beautifully made instruments, simply constructed and able to produce a good sound relatively easily invite one to touch and explore them. Their size and portability is a factor in making them accessible to and playable by a patient at home, perhaps bedbound, and restricted by a range of physical disability. A person's curiosity and wonder can help overcome self-consciousness. Trying out a 'new' instrument, not met before, can have refreshing consequences when there may not be outside standards to fall short of.

Instruments aside, many people are reluctant to give voice but may sing or hum along to well-known or favourite songs or join in a chorus; even tapping on the table in time or breathing with the pulse of the music is a choice to be part of the creative flow.

Meeting patients

How do I meet patients? Nurses and social workers from the home care teams make referrals. Sometimes patients and their families expressly wish for some input of a musical nature and sometimes a referral is made because of the vaguest of musical connections with a patient. I need to address the question of how I am to describe myself so that team members have some useful information to offer families and patients. Yet it is only when I meet patients that there is any clarity about what is appropriate. Already, I am introduced as an art or music therapist and this is misleading. For the moment, I have decided to let myself be described as 'a member of the arts team' but make care team members aware that the work I am doing is not limited to music, and patients do not need to have it as part of their background.

Keith was a man in his forties with a brain tumour who was referred to me. He had an interest in music and his family ran a music shop. He was also of an extremely anxious nature and it was felt that some kind of musical interaction might help him to relax. He was a single man and unable to live independently, so he was currently in a nursing home; there was a considerable age difference between him and other residents. He was unable to use his left side and spent his time either in bed or sitting in a chair, supported by cushions. When staff were available he might sometimes be wheelchaired into the garden. I went to visit him and decided to take my flute and a hammer dulcimer with the idea that he might be able to explore the strings of the dulcimer with his fingers or hammers and we might create some music together. Both instruments are portable and accessible and beautifully made, good to touch, potentially pleasant and calming in their sound and at least interesting topics of conversation.

Keith was talkative, shy, interested but ill at ease; he hopped from subject to subject hurriedly and wasn't comfortable with silence. He was interested in the dulcimer as an ancestor of the piano and asked lots of questions. He was wary of playing and tentative, preferring to talk rather than do or be. I sensed that my encouragement to play was increasing his anxiety. I decided to play a slow tune on the wooden flute and suggested he listened. It was a permission he seemed to need because he closed his eyes and went quiet and sat back in his chair. Other tunes followed. He appeared to take the music as sound massage. I began to treat it as such and improvised around themes based on the movement of his fingers of his right hand, focusing sometimes on his left arm which he could no longer use. He asked about the names of the tunes; if it was an improvisation we would consider appropriate names.

I reflected on whether my visit had been successful. I had hoped that there would have been more mutuality in our music making but realised that starting with this instrument by playing together demanded too much from him and amplified his anxiety. I would have to start more simply next time, perhaps using a drum or a bell. He had embraced the experience of the flute music positively and while he wanted to know about the instrument, the science and the facts, how it worked and where the music came from, he also allowed himself to be quiet and surrender to the atmosphere created by its sound. There had been warmth and humour in our exchanges; he was interested in my visiting again.

In further visits Keith was less able to play himself, but wanted to listen to the flute and liked it being played for him. It has been a ritual for us that allows us to talk in a reflective way, interspersed with playing, and occasionally distracting from the physical discomfort that was beginning to fill his days. It was something we shared. He had some favourite tunes, which he liked to revisit. Most of all, it allowed us to be together in a gentle way without talking too much. On reflection, I realise that my playing was not a 'performance'; I was not playing 'the entertainer' but providing the kind of communication that helped him to get beyond words.

Rachel was at first reluctant to accept a visit from me. A woman in her eighties living alone, she had become low in spirits and wary of unfamiliar faces. I arranged to visit with a community nurse specialist (CNS), whom she was used to seeing and we met at last. She talked for an hour and a half in spite of her need for oxygen. Clearly, she was a natural extrovert and drew energy from meeting other people. She wanted to talk about her life and loved joking.

In her childhood, she had sung round the piano with her sisters so the opportunity to sing brought back some of her life and evoked many memories. One song in particular was very significant for her because her husband had sung it during their courtship during the Blackout in the east end of London in the Second World War. She couldn't quite remember the whole melody but I was able to find it on the internet, a popular song from a 1940 film, and we put it back together and sang it at every visit. I recorded her singing it with some of the stories that she told about her and her husband's 'Blackout' meeting.

A complication with Rachel's illness brought her into the hospice for a number of weeks and we were able to continue with our music making. She was keen to include the other patients who shared her bay and the singing of fondly remembered songs stimulated the contact between the women and led to a lot of sharing about themselves. Rachel's capacity for remembering the words of songs was remarkable and contributed life and energy to the group and to our transactions. I became aware that the songs of Dean Martin, Nat King Cole and others were the emotional currency of a generation. I took some of them with me to my extended family's annual gathering that included people from my parents' generation. It was noticeable how much the community united in singing them; they brought back happy memories.

Rachel has tried a number of times to return home to live, but her care needs mean that she needed the support of a nursing home. During this confusing, disorientating time our regular singing and chatting sessions were familiar and regular. It has underlined for me the importance of being committed as a member of her community.

Henry was a man in his eighties with cancer, referred to me as someone who seemed to be very depressed; he had stopped talking even to his wife. He had had an interest in classical music and might benefit from a visit. His wife met me at the door and said he was in bed and in poor form, but that I was welcome to meet him. Both at one time had made regular visits to the opera and we were able to share our interest in such music as well as theatre in general. Henry talked very little. He responded mostly in monosyllables but made good eye contact with me. I was not sure whether he was reluctant, perhaps too fed up, to speak or unable to find the words. He sometimes began a long sentence in response to a question, but was unable to supply a main clause or subject. I felt that his word-finding skills were impaired through his illness and that his hearing and understanding certainly were not. We agreed that I would continue to visit.

After a few visits in which we talked slightly disjointedly or sat silently, I arrived with my flute and a bowl-harp, a carved wooden bowl strung with a dozen strings, beautiful to look at, to touch and to hear. I felt that since conversation was difficult we might be able to share some music. The introduction of some new medication had lightened Henry's mood and he examined the bowl with interest. His fingers wandered over the carved elm and he touched the strings; then rested his fingers on the side of the bowl, lost in his thoughts. Occasionally he moved back to the strings and plucked one or two and I was able to respond on other strings or on my flute. Octaves and unisons. It felt like we were tuning in to each other as well as exploring the bowl that lay between us. Our exchange of sounds was simply that. It was an acknowledgement of each other, respectful and dignified. I'm not sure what was 'said' but I have a real sense that we met.

Raising awareness

The other aspect of my role at St Christopher's involves raising awareness in the community of the hospice's work, helping to break down taboos around death and dying. I remember from my own experience as a child in the 1950s and 1960s the cultural barriers put in the way of a natural experience of death. I had been prevented from attending the funeral of a favourite grandfather who had always shared our family home because of the anxiety that it might be upsetting for me. I remembered too the experience of so many learning disabled people who were kept away from those family occasions, because it was feared they would not understand or be upset.

When I arrived at the hospice a project was already being planned to introduce a group of school children to St Christopher's (see Chapter 2 for a discussion of the management and development of this project). It followed on from a project with the same school last year; the school had seen the benefit for the children and wanted the next group of 9–10-year-old pupils to have the same opportunity.

We had several aims in bringing patients, staff and school children together. As well as to publicising the hospice's work, we wanted to reduce anxiety in the school community and in children's families around the subject of illness, death and dying; to facilitate mutual acknowledgement and appreciation of youth, age, curiosity and life experience and the struggles of life and to explore a variety of artistic media.

The project would involve a visit to the hospice by the school children, staff, some parents and teaching assistants, to see some of the facilities and meet some of the patients using the day unit. Then, arts team members would work with the children back at school for two successive Wednesdays. The project would conclude with a further visit to the hospice in which the arts team and the students would share some of their work with the patients and school and hospice staff.

My two colleagues, both visual artists, and I, planned the two school days taking the theme of 'journey'; we would explore together the way human lives are journeys, with beginnings, twists and turns, ups and downs, and ends. We would share and create stories using words, visual images and music. We planned to have stories to show and to say and songs to sing when we returned to the hospice on the last day of the project. There was good creative flow between us as we prepared the themes; later we took turns to 'animate' the process of informing and preparing the group to work. We shared questions too. How might we incorporate the issues raised by the children's visit to the hospice? How directive must we be in facilitating the children's story making? We concluded that the children must go where they wanted to go with their stories. We would suggest 'gifts' and 'challenges' they might want to use. We saw the importance of approaching the subject of living with terminal illness and death in an oblique way, leaving the children free to choose to incorporate their thoughts and feelings about their visit to the hospice into the creative work.

We worked intensively together over two days. The children teemed with ideas, images, characters and situations. They worked in groups and collaborated well. They negotiated the sharing of tasks and making decisions about what ideas to include and develop. Choosing faces of anonymous people cut from magazines, the children gave them names and life stories. We asked them to tell the journeys of their lives in words and pictures. They chose particular joys and sorrows that either illuminated or overshadowed their characters' lives. Some of their creations inhabited the bizarre worlds of internet games, gadget-bound and violent, locked in titanic struggles. Others dealt with relationship break-up, the burden of celebrity, family jealousies and illness, loneliness and the experience of war. We decided to incorporate many of the stories into a book which we could show on our return visit to the hospice and it became a collection of laminated pages with sequences of faces, drawings, narratives and poems. We used a simple writing frame to structure the poems and again these were collaborations of groups of children. We also rehearsed a travelling song by Sidney Carter and created a song called 'What will You Bring?' (to the tune 'We are Sailing' by Rod Stewart) as part of a ritual in which people are invited to list a few of the special things they would want to have 'at their journey's end':

> What will you bring? What will you bring
> As we walk down to the shore?
> What will you bring when the time comes
> When we walk down to the shore?
>
> I'll bring......................
> I'll bring....................
> I'll bring......................
> When we walk down to the shore.

At the end of the second day in school, parents were invited to join their children in the classroom and we shared some of the work we had been engaged in and invited questions and comments. Six children brought family representatives: 20 per cent of the class. They were clearly proud of the work their children were doing, and moved by the seriousness of their attitude. Some of them shared anxieties they had had about their children being involved in such a project.

On the fourth day of the project, children and parents met patients and staff in the chapel at St Christopher's. With a slide-show of photographs of the children at work on the project showing in the background, the children read out their poems. We sang our songs and some children shared their thoughts about what the experience had been like for them. Some of the patients responded with gratitude, appreciation and humour. The afternoon ended with a tea party. On the following day, we repeated the presentation at school assembly with the whole school and many parents present.

In evaluating the project I was struck by how much of an experiment it was and that everyone involved had some anxiety about what it might bring. It was a challenge for patients to present themselves in a public arena and take direct questions about their experience of the hospice from children. The children were coming into an unfamiliar environment where they knew there were people who were terminally ill. Here are some of their comments written anonymously:

> 'I felt nervous but when I got used to it I liked it.'

> 'I felt more happier after I realised that death is not a scary thing. Although I felt sad leaving all the people there.'

> 'I felt kind of nervous and scared because I thought it was going to be upsetting…'

> 'A bit scared because people are sick and I feel sad for them.'

> ' I felt very happy and proud when we showed our work to the whole school because everyone loved it and at the end I didn't feel scared any more and I felt like they were one of us.'

> 'I felt like you could be yourself and have loads of fun.'

Some patients told me how much they liked the liveliness and energy of the children around them. Parents of children connected with patients; the tea party had the atmosphere of people at the start of a relationship. I noticed a group of boys who had created a fictional life story about a man who had bad memories of his time as a soldier. They were engaged in conversation with an elderly patient who was under the impression that this man was actually one of their grandfathers. He seemed to make a connection between the fictional 'grandfather's' experience and his own experience of Normandy on D-Day. His real desire to tell them about his war story was as clear as their great hunger to hear it. Their story touched such a universal chord that when the same group of boys shared it at school assembly a child in the audience spontaneously called out, 'I know that man'.

The creation of fictional stories allowed the children to explore some of the difficult issues that human beings encounter in their lives. Some of these included end-of-life themes such as loneliness, isolation, the pain and disability of illness and more existential, spiritual themes such as 'What is the value or meaning of my life?' through the consideration both of war trauma and of celebrity.

The project had been a meeting place, an interface where 'death is not a scary thing' has become more possible through actual meetings between children and terminally ill people and through the children's imaginative journeys. A shared imaginative meeting and journey was possible, in which patient and child had the possibility of creating together. Real encounters can be challenging, but life-affirming and life-giving.

This became the focus of our planning for the next school project, again with a primary school where a relationship had begun with St Christopher's the previous year. We wanted both children and patients to have more time together and have the possibility of more creative interaction.

My colleagues suggested making masks. A group of patients would make the basic shapes using *papier mâché* over balloons then halving them and then together with the children painting them so there was a mask for each child. The familiar theatre ikon of the joyful/melancholy masks put me in mind of some lines of William Blake in his 'Auguries of Innocence':

> It is right it should be so;
> Man was made for joy and woe;
> And when this we rightly know,
> Through the world we safely go.
>
> Joy and woe are woven fine,
> A clothing for the soul divine.
> Under every grief and pine
> Runs a joy with silken twine.

I thought this would be an important theme to explore in the context of the mask making and might lead us into creative writing and music making. It was necessary for practical reasons to divide the group of 30 schoolchildren into two groups of 15, one group at a time would work with the patients on the masks in the day centre, while I worked with the others back at school.

Even though an important aim of this project was to have patients and children working together, it was still important for the children to be working together on a theme and presenting it to an audience that includes patients. As with the children in the first project, it might help them to process their experience of visiting the hospice and meeting patients both consciously and through the imagination. It is a familiar way of working in primary schools: there is a goal and an outcome. The presentation is given as a gift and there is the opportunity for their achievements and efforts to be acknowledged. Choosing an 'interesting activity' can seem to be just 'an excuse' to bring people together. It can do more. Enjoyment can be thought-provoking, leading to reflection and various levels of acknowledgement of the crucial transitions that both children and people in the final stages of their lives are making.

Again the project began with a visit to the hospice; then two days of either hospice-based or school-based activities, culminating in an afternoon of presentation and tea in the hospice day centre. The school also wanted to host an assembly about the project and invite patients.

With the first school-based group we had no masks to work with, because they had not made them yet, so we created a series of improvised musical pieces culminating in the traditional gospel song: 'Nobody Knows the Trouble I Seen' exploring the concept of 'woe'. Then we created another sequence which led to the singing and playing of the Beatles' song: 'Good Day, Sunshine' as a way of expressing joy. There was a strong tradition of music in the school and a good range of instruments to choose from and a great eagerness on the part of the children to experiment.

The second day's work revolved around the masks that the children had made with patients the previous week. We paid great respect to the masks themselves, as is the tradition, and explored using them with movement, characterisation and improvised music. The children were inventive, physically eloquent, and by turns solemn and irreverent behind their masks. The masks had their limitations. They had no eyes and no easy way of fixing them to the face. There was time to reflect on the Blake poem and the children introduced some important ideas – the pattern of ups and downs that can be recognised in our lives – the wheel of fortune – and the consideration that we as human beings are not perfect.

The presentation took place in a garden pavilion; it was crammed with children, masks, parents and some patients although not many were able to be there, as sometimes happens. The programme included music, songs, poems and displays of the masks through simple sketches. There was a cosy, chaotic informality about the occasion and opportunities to meet and talk. I was struck by the contrast with the first day when the children sat there, stiff, anxious and still. A similar presentation took place at school and two of the patients were able to attend. It was noticeable how many of the children had made cards to send to patients they had spent time with at the day unit; evidence of good connections made.

The class teacher told me that the previous Year 5 pupils, aged 9 to 10 year olds who had taken part in the first St Christopher's project wrote about their primary school experience before leaving to go on to their secondary schools. Many of them mentioned their encounter with St Christopher's as their most abiding memory.

Conclusion

As I review my first few months as an artist in palliative care, I am aware of how much I am being challenged, as an artist, to respond imaginatively, to find 'ways in' to music making, to writing, image making, that encourage, inspire and invite. Being patient and accepting of the difficulties and frustrations caused by the effect of illness in a person's life is important, as is being an opportunist in seizing the moment to make a creative intervention; it might never happen again. It was important to record Rachel singing the song her husband sang her when they were courting, even though she had forgotten some of it because by the time I had found the complete song she was not well enough to sing it. How important too to reflect on what has happened in sessions with patients in all their details. I think of Paul, who was referred to me as someone who wanted to write. When I met him, he just wanted to talk about football and his memories of his life as a football supporter. I was very happy to share that with him and, when I listened to the recording I had made, I realised his football experiences were a metaphor for the whole of his life and he was reflecting in my presence on his meaning and value and worth as a man. It was a privilege to witness that.

I realise too how important it is to let the nurses in the home care teams know the kinds of things I am doing so that they can imagine some of the possibilities for the patients they meet every day.

I began this reflection with many questions. Of course they reveal my insecurities as I stand on the threshold of new responsibilities, but behind that they touch on my own fear of death. The questions about language and communication will always be important. I find that good communication between everyone in the patient's caring community is crucial in best serving their needs.

In one's final illness there may be many different challenges when help from medical staff for pain relief, symptom control, dietary support, physiotherapy, household aids, spiritual and psychological care, social work input to help with economic and personal affairs can make significant contributions to the quality of our lives while never obscuring our individual humanity. I see that the artist can have a place there too. Through collaboration in the world of music, metaphor and image he can help to re-member and witness the richness and mysterious value of each person's life.

13 Music Therapy in the Community

Tamsin Dives

Why music therapy at the end of life?

Because people are living much longer these days we need to think more creatively about how we care for older people. Their health needs and care contexts are many and varied and this throws up exciting and challenging issues which we, as therapists, should consider. In old age, many people review and evaluate their life (Ronaldson 1997). There is a great need for supportive emotional care as the 'meaning of life' perhaps overrides physical needs. Older people often have to adapt to a rapid succession of changes, many associated with loss. Palliative care seeks to integrate all domains of supportive care: physical, psychological, existential and spiritual. Music therapy can help to meet some of these needs. It can help maximise and enhance quality of life.

St Christopher's Hospice decided to set up an outreach project resourcing local care homes to provide a course of music therapy, hoping that, eventually, homes would establish and fund music therapy for themselves. The idea behind this was to extend the care currently available to patients at St Christopher's to other people living in the local community, nearing the end of their life. As music therapist, I have recently joined the St Christopher's arts team and have taken on the work of this outreach project. One day a week, I visit residential homes, running groups and some one-to-one sessions. Two of the homes are for older people and I visit one home for adults who require long-term, permanent care.

Setting up

A colleague made the initial contact with care homes local to the community of St Christopher's. She sent out a letter explaining what St Christopher's could provide and offered three free introductory sessions to any home interested.

The three sessions took place over three consecutive weeks. The D'Oyly Carte Charitable Trust funded these introductory sessions, supporting the hospice's aim to introduce the potential of group music therapy to care homes.

Of ten local care homes contacted, five chose to receive these initial sessions. The first session informed the staff about the potential of group music therapy. It included a brief presentation using recordings of work with people in similar situations to the residents of the home. It also included some discussion about who might best benefit from group music therapy. She suggested that it might benefit people who:

- have limited other means of interaction, communication and spontaneity
- have low mood, low motivation
- have few outlets for emotional expression of difficult feelings
- are unwilling to engage in more prescriptive therapies such as speech and language therapy or physiotherapy
- are socially isolated in the care setting
- are emotionally isolated from other residents
- find one-to-one stimulation too intense.

The first session also offered a forum for music therapist and staff to consider together how they might best support residents during a session, for example:

- Explore ways of helping individuals to play instruments without doing it for them and give them examples of how to give physical support. For instance, I have sometimes observed that staff, with the best will in the world, are so keen for the clients to participate that they will almost 'play' the instrument for the client. To examine and suggest ways of being supportive in an unobtrusive way before music therapy sessions commence is invaluable.

- Discuss how the residents might use the 'therapy' time; that it's all right for residents to have a choice about how they participate; they might perhaps wish to remain quiet during a session.

- Offer an opportunity for staff to participate in some group music making themselves. This gave staff an immediate impression of the potential of group music therapy.

Care home staff and the therapist chose specific residents to take part in the two following group sessions. When the sessions took place, staff attended and were able to observe the responses of the group. Nineteen members of care home staff attended the teaching sessions and thirteen members of staff observed group music therapy sessions. There were, overall, a total of 52 patient contacts in the group music therapy sessions.

The staff were asked for their observations of the residents during and following the music therapy sessions and any impact the session had had on themselves, either directly or indirectly. Responses about communication and participation were as follows:

- Instead of saying 'No, not today', G participated.

- To see E responding like that! Normally she refuses and if you ask her twice she shouts, but she did play the instruments at the beginning of the session last week and this week she sang a bit.

- And M came out of his room! He hasn't been out of his room in ages.

- The music session seemed to bring them together.

- S sang 'Hello' to you on his own. He was responding to you. You were at his level.

- It's hard to tell if J responds but I really think he did: his eyes lit up.

Staff also remarked on residents' mood and self-confidence.

- J wished he'd been able to come down last week. He was really upset before he came down but then did you see the smile on his face by the end of the session?

- G hasn't sworn half as much since the first session last week. She used to love music. I think it's going in.

- B was more aware in the second session. She's been talking about the first session. She enjoyed it.

- Sometimes in the week since the first session, A's still been anxious but she's much calmer in herself. She's been laughing more. I think it's proved to her that she can still do things. Usually she's said 'I can't, I can't'. She's been much less tearful and able to calm herself when you might tell her something that before might have been distressing.

- W seemed more confident in the second session and the day after the first session last week, he got out his harmonica and played all morning. It's amazing. I can't believe it.

They also commented on whether relatives, other residents and staff had seen any changes in those who had received music therapy.

- E used to speak but she had stopped except for saying 'yes, yes, yes'. She had stopped feeding herself too. But since the music therapy session last week, I don't know whether it's a coincidence but she said her son's name when he visited and when I asked her how she was feeling she said 'Better'. It's only single words but it's like she's trying to communicate. Also one of the nurses left her breakfast in front of her and when she came back E had started to eat. Her son has seen a difference in her and is thrilled. He went to the residents' and relatives' association meeting and said how thrilled he was.

- A was a different woman since the music therapy session last week. Her husband noticed a difference. Usually she doesn't really join in; she just sits on the sofa. This week though, since the first session, when her husband visited her she went straight to the front door to meet him and tried to tell him about the music session. She's starting to join in other activities and mix with other residents and they're starting to make an effort to understand her speech.

On being present at the group music therapy sessions staff commented:

- I was dubious at first, but having seen it, I got quite tearful watching E, seeing you work your magic.

- I learnt a lot watching the session. It's broadened my horizons knowing that music can communicate, not necessarily only words.

- It was good to see it in practice.

- I can see it changing them, making them more sociable.

Staff saw the benefits and were keen for the work to continue. I was then employed to carry on this work, leaving my colleague free to continue practising music therapy on the St Christopher's site and with St Christopher's patients in the community.

Developing the programme

I started working in three homes, with two other homes interested in receiving a block of music therapy as soon as it can be arranged. Sessions have been booked in blocks of six with an opportunity to review the work with staff after the sixth session. This gives us the possibility of making changes within the group if appropriate. It's also a valuable focus for dialogue and feedback about the work. So far in my work at the homes the group members have remained consistent and the homes are committed to long-term projects.

I take with me a collection of instruments, percussion, tuned and untuned, all very easy to use. Some have been specifically adapted for those who might otherwise find them difficult to play. I also have a guitar and electronic keyboard. During the sessions, residents explore improvised music making and other musical activities. They use their voices with or without words depending on their capacity, what they feel they would like to do. We sing familiar songs and make up new ones.

The groups I run have been closed. Residents are encouraged not to drop in and out. It's available for the same group members each week and there seems a real commitment from residents to attend. They value this regular space. The sessions are 45 minutes long and happen at the same time each week. Each home has a different style about it and I find I have to be very flexible. Sometimes it takes a while to collect people together. Residents occasionally feel confused and disorientated and need time to settle before a session begins.

The work

The group I have worked with longest are mainly in their nineties. All are wheelchair-bound and have a variety of diagnoses. Of the regular members, two are in the later stages of dementia, one has learning disabilities and two are sprightly. So there is a mix of those who can engage in lively conversation together with those who can't. To begin with, I wondered whether this was a good idea. How, in a space especially for them, could I work with the verbal and non-verbal together? But, of course, music does not require people to use words.

These residents are isolated during the day spending a large proportion of their day in their rooms. This is largely due to the layout of the home. It's difficult to get to the lounge area and the corridors are long and narrow, stretching off in different directions. One particular group member is choosing to spend more and more time alone during her week; however, she has chosen to come to music therapy. She seems to find it alarming to be with other people, so this is a rare and challenging opportunity to be with others. Perhaps because music therapy offers a space where words don't have to be used, she is able to accept challenge, whereas in other aspects of her life she feels she must be more cautious.

Although this is the most frail group I am involved with, it is quite lively. A great deal of free improvisation takes place. They seem to enjoy spontaneous music making and I am often surprised how sustained their playing is and also by the 'tempo' of the music created. We sing together too, and this is often followed by lots of chatter and sharing of memories. There is talk of loved ones and happy times but also individuals express their frustration and sadness. During a conversation after singing 'Daisy Daisy, Give me Your Answer Do' one resident remembered sitting on the handlebars of her boyfriend's bike coming home from a date; another talked of riding a tandem through leafy lanes in Kent.

One of the group members who has dementia communicates only in a 'singsong' way. His words are jumbled. It's sometimes very hard to get a sense of what he's saying, but every time I've met him, he has very clearly told me that all his family are dead. He constantly mentions his mother too. He's physically very frail and often left alone as he can be very aggressive; this has worsened with his dementia. He was a chemist and the staff remember him as a real gentleman, a charmer. The group spends much of the session singing together, he sings along joining us in spirit and energy but not with words and melody. Everyone welcomes his contributions and I hope that his lively engagement is satisfying to him. His mood certainly becomes brighter. At other times, I improvise along with him. I can get a real sense of his personality by the way he sings. It's warm, witty and colourful. We swoop up and down together, sharing notes, sharing space. It's possible to 'meet' with him. Singing is a secure and valid way for him to be with someone else; it validates his humanity. It also gives him a place to be active and independent, something hard to achieve in his environment.

Growing old is something most people hope to experience. Working with older people, many personal emotional issues emerge for the therapist. We become aware of our own mortality. That frail old person could be me, will be me. We consider our parents; do we feel guilty at the level of our involvement in their lives? Are we fearful for our own final years? Might we end up like this? Who will look after us, when other family members can't?

I'm suggesting that there is a different sort of emotional involvement for people who work with this particular client group, which puts a very particular sort of pressure on the carers of older people. This might be especially relevant in Western society where in many instances the idea of care for the extended family has disappeared. We tend to categorise the elderly; distancing ourselves from them by labelling them as either 'revered or respected' or 'grumpy and difficult'. Is there a resistance to working with frail, elderly people?

Music therapy can facilitate thinking about this client group. It will encourage carers to think of older people as individuals, spiritual beings who are still growing and evolving.

Music on the move

There are potential difficulties for the visiting therapist to the care home. A therapy space needs to be found where privacy and intimacy can be respected. Often this is a space shared by many professional teams and this can be confusing for the client.

I take my instruments around with me and after I leave at the end of a session all that is left in the home is a memory of an event or perhaps not even that, perhaps nothing tangible to relate to.

So I feel a great responsibility to 'make, hold and carry' the therapeutic space. A 'do not disturb' sign goes on the door, but that is sometimes ignored. Each time I visit the home, I try to make some form of contact with staff and residents alike, whether it's a nod, smile or chat; this makes me feel more comfortable. Visiting these homes for a short burst and then moving on somewhere else, it is difficult for me to get a sense of being part of a team. Nurses and staff are perhaps more concerned with the physical needs of residents, whereas I get caught up in their emotional needs. And how do I pass across to the staff my impressions of the music therapy sessions?

Understandably there is the potential for the 'nomadic' therapist to become the target of negative feeling. We're not working there day in, day out. We can walk away, it seems. It is important to remind people that the therapist is not an entertainer or performer, but is creating a forum for therapeutic work.

I wonder what I symbolise to the staff? I think that for some of them there is a fear that I might be judgemental of the way they are managing. Some care homes have received a bad press in recent years. Indeed there is a variety of care, some better than others. On the same day I might visit places with a different working ethos, quality of care and standard of building. I need to have a very clear sense of my own working ethos. One of the hazards of being a visitor is that I am a useful ear for staff with issues and can leave, burdened with their frustrations – not properly my concern.

Each environment I work in has a very different quality about it. Each group is particular with specific dynamics and requirements. Each organisation has asked for a different type of feedback. With one home I have a very fluid easy relationship with the manager and I feel that the feedback from sessions has been informative and helped her to think of individuals in a different way. Her openness affects the ethos of the whole building. The nurses are interested and interesting. One nurse wondered if her presence in the group was affecting one resident's ability to access the music therapy, although she's always been a very flexible and supportive helper. She suggested she withdrew and she was right. The resident grew a little in confidence and started to engage more with the music.

Another of my experiences is of a residential care home for adults of all ages. The atmosphere is vibrant and there is considerable interest in alternative/holistic approaches to care. The staff are young and energetic. It's a noisy place full of chatter, laughter and positive bustle. It's very much a place for the living. The therapy space however has a very different energy. Here many difficult emotions are released, which are perhaps hard to voice elsewhere in the home.

Not all experiences in homes have been so fruitful. One has to have courage in the face of less than helpful conditions.

I also do some one-to-one work with residents in their rooms. Two of these are bedbound. Although they are both limited physically, a great deal happens in these sessions. One resident communicates with his eyes; another, a lady, with little physical movement, joins me as I sing by sticking her tongue out in time to the music. Behind closed doors another talks of the difficulties he has with 'fitting in'.

Support

Visiting more than one home a day and then driving back I often find it hard to hold in my head what has happened during the day. I make notes at each home and I also make more comprehensive notes back at St Christopher's. I also record a mini-disk of each session. In moving on to a different workplace, there's the danger of becoming disconnected from where you have just been. 'Not belonging' is perhaps a problem when you are doing a lot of outreach work. It's good to get back to the base; my colleague is always available to talk things through. St Christopher's has a dynamic and wide-ranging arts therapy team. The team has begun to meet regularly to discuss different aspects of their work, which has proved enormously fruitful and supportive. Whatever the medium therapy work is rooted in, the same issues seem to come up. It's important to me to feel I'm a part of the hospice too. I also regularly have invaluable supervision.

The groups

One of the groups I run has six regular members, four women and two men. All are in their mid-forties and all the group members are wheelchair-bound. I'd like to talk about one of the men whom I shall call Sam. He comes from an African country. Because of his injuries he has lost the use of his voice and has restricted use of one arm. He is highly educated and a devout Muslim. His injuries mean he has a very limited way of expressing himself and he often appears isolated. The women in this group are verbally articulate and assured and the talk during the sessions is often quite fiery. Sam is part of the group and listens and understands but can't join in the banter. It's not surprising that, for several weeks, Sam chose to play the drum during every session, refusing any other instrument offered. This allowed him to play across conversation and music, often continuing to play after everyone else had stopped. It was as if, in his isolation, he had forgotten he could be part of a group. His beating drum was a powerful way to make his presence felt. However, as the weeks have gone by, Sam's playing has relaxed, it's not so erratic, he seems to listen to what other members are doing and they've begun to listen to him too.

Once, in an improvised piece, I was singing while playing the guitar. Everyone had a percussion instrument and I was leaving space for individuals to contribute as and when they wanted. Sam, who I had never heard make a sound, started to sing back to me, copying my rhythms and at the right pitch. He laughed as we 'turn took' together. We always start our session with an improvised 'Hello' song. The members of the group have always chosen to sing as well and Sam now vocalises when I sing 'Hello' to him. He has also relinquished his drum and chooses to play more melodic instruments. Because words are not necessary in this forum, it is a valuable place for Sam, because he is able to be self-expressive and interact with others without having to use words.

In another group I run, conversation outweighs music making. It's as if the music is a catalyst for thoughts. One particular lady, I'll call her Eve, is very confused. She sits and cries silently. 'I am a *real* musician,' she says. 'You don't understand, I'm a *real* musician; I used to play the organ.' She won't play any instruments but if we sing she eventually joins in. She talks colourfully about music making when she was a young woman but can't remember the names of her children. She describes herself as 'having gone, I just live'. She's seems to have always had a deep emotional connection to music and I'm sure the sessions are painful because they remind her of what she has lost. Nevertheless, she has a lot she wants to say and somehow the musical environment gives her a platform to do this – *and* she keeps coming back.

Another lady in this group is in the advanced stages of Parkinson's disease. Her voice is weak and she has a severe tremor. I've noticed that if I give her a shaker to play her tremor seems to relax. She is able to play quite rhythmically and seems much more in control of her movements. She likes to sing the old songs and talks of her husband who has died. 'I can see him so clearly, it's been three years since he died and I just can't get over it,' she says. 'The music really helps.'

There's also a lot of fun too. Jeff with a voice like Mario Lanza and a twinkle in his eye sings rude words to the old music hall song 'After the Ball is Over'. Everyone laughs.

Conclusion

As I pass through different institutions, I've realised that one of the most important qualities to have for this work is flexibility. You never quite know how things are going to be. Therefore, I think it's helpful to have a robust outlook, to be self-reliant but it's also important to find allies amongst your staff to enable you to do your best work. You need a sense of the dynamics of each particular work place.

I come away from the work feeling there is a spirit ripened by the passage of years in many older people. These are powerful people with much to say. Music can give them a voice, and sharing in music stimulates meaningful memories and supports emotional expression. It gives the elderly a forum to make choices and decisions at a time when their outlooks are limited. Music can be a source of great comfort in the last phase of life providing something creative, something of worth and something to look forward to.

14 Music and Music Therapy at St Christopher's Hospice – An Evaluation Study

Abi Gill

Introduction

I was the first person employed as a music therapist at St Christopher's Hospice, and was asked not only to provide music therapy sessions, but also to help bring music into the life of the hospice as a whole. I worked for two days a week on-site, across the day unit and the wards, and for one further day with patients in their homes and care homes. As the service developed, I was asked to find a way to evaluate the music therapy sessions and other musical events that took place on-site. Independent researchers conducted a separate evaluation study into music therapy and art sessions that took place in community settings.

This chapter will summarise some of the existing literature describing music therapy work in palliative care, and then describe the results of the study at St Christopher's.

Music and music therapy in palliative care

There is a relatively small but growing body of literature discussing the use of music therapy in the specialist palliative care of adult patients. This includes music therapists' descriptions of work with patients (Hartley 2001; Hogan 2003; O'Callaghan 1996) and descriptions of a range of techniques used in sessions, including co-improvisation, song writing and musical life reviews (Hogan 2003; Munro in Magee 2000). Some therapists have described theoretical concepts that guide them in their work with palliative care patients (Salmon 2001).

These authors describe the benefits that they have seen music therapy sessions bring to patients, carers, friends and family members, including a reduction in anxiety and isolation, the alleviation of pain and an increased sense of empowerment for patients. Sessions may also provide a focus for family visits, where visitors may see the patient unusually active and enjoying themselves whilst participating in making music. Some therapists have described a broader use of music in a hospice setting, including the use of live and recorded music to alleviate specific difficulties faced by palliative care patients, such as chronic pain (O'Callaghan 1996).

Music therapy at St Christopher's

The evaluation took place over nine months, beginning 18 months after I started working at the hospice. During this period, I received 26 referrals to music therapy. A total of 81 sessions took place, most patients receiving between one and five sessions but with a few having up to 17 weekly sessions. Most patients continued coming to sessions for the time they remained under the care of St Christopher's. In the case of several referrals on the inpatient unit (IPU), the patient died before a first session was possible. This was usually due to a combination of my working only two days a week on-site and a rapid, unexpected deterioration in some patients' health.

Most music therapy sessions took place in the music room, with eight sessions taking place at the bedside on the ward and five taking place in other parts of the hospice. One patient came to sessions whilst an inpatient, and was then discharged to a nursing home. We continued to have sessions at the care home, to which his 12-year-old son also came. When this man died quite suddenly, I subsequently worked on-site with his son, offering support in bereavement.

Most sessions took place on a one-to-one basis, although some also involved the patient's family and friends. Sessions on the ward sometimes involved other patients and visitors in the bay. Referrals were almost equal in number for male and female patients. Eighteen were aged between 50 and 80, four were in their eighties and three in their forties. Only one referral was for a patient younger than 40. Most patients referred were of a white British background, with four referrals being for patients belonging to a minority ethnic group. Most of those indicating a religious affiliation belonged to a Christian denomination. Twenty-one of the 26 referrals were for patients who were staying on the wards, although not all of these were made by ward staff. Other staff referring patients on the ward included the Director of the Creative Living Centre, a member of the complementary therapy team and a member of Hospice at Home staff. One inpatient asked to come to sessions himself, and the husband of another inpatient requested some live music to be played at his wife's bedside. Referrals for patients attending the day unit were mostly made by the day unit nursing team.

Of the 26 referrals, most patients had a diagnosis of malignant disease, most commonly cancer of the breast, lung or prostate; three were living with non-malignant disease. Reasons for referral included raising confidence and self-esteem, improving mood and lowering anxiety, increasing social contact, acting as a non-verbal means of communication, and because of the patient's love of music. Some referrers were less specific: those who referred a patient for general stimulation and engagement in activity or for a form of one-to-one therapeutic input, or those who felt there was something missing from the patient's care and wondered whether music therapy might help. A small number of referrals were for a patient and their family to enjoy an activity together at the bedside, one that was light-hearted and focused on something other than the patient's illness.

Patients used their sessions in a variety of ways. Forty-five sessions involved the patient and therapist improvising together, using singing and melodic and non-melodic percussion. In 19 sessions the patient learned and practised a familiar tune on an instrument, most commonly the piano. Many sessions also involved my accompanying patients as they sang songs that were familiar and special to them, or patients learning new songs of a particular style. Several sessions involved patients writing a song of their own. With one patient, I sat and listened to classical music CDs. Another asked for vocal exercises to help retrieve his former singing voice. We worked on these exercises in sessions, and he took them home with him, enjoying 'practising' them with his young grandson. Some patients talked about their enjoyment of music, and some used the time to talk about non-music-related issues that were important to them or situations that they were finding difficult.

Another patient asked me to improvise music in particular styles, to which she invented stories and songs. I worked with this woman over a number of months, both when she came to the day unit, and when she was admitted to the ward. One week, she was feeling very unwell and preferred to rest alone, but asked that I go to the music room and 'play music for her', which I did. In my improvising, I included a few lines from melodies we had learnt and enjoyed together, as well as some phrases that recalled music we had improvised. I recorded the session and later asked her if she would like to hear what I had played. As we listened, she recognised the parts that were references to sessions we had had together. As she listened to a part that recalled music in which she had sung in an unusually open and vulnerable way, she described this as 'her tune'. She later she told me that she might have part of the recording played at her funeral.

There were other times when patients declined sessions, and did not ask that I play for them. For the most part this was due to their feeling tired or in pain; sometimes it was because they had promised to take part in another activity at that time. When this happened, if the patient wanted and if I was able, we arranged another time for the session.

Exploring patient and carer experiences in music therapy sessions

During the evaluation period, I invited each patient who had attended more than three music therapy sessions to take part in an informal interview. I did not approach for interview patients whom the multi-professional team thought were not cognitively able to give informed consent, or who were seen to be in significant distress. A music therapy colleague, who was not a member of staff at the hospice, carried out the interviews. He used a series of questions to prompt the interviewee to describe their experiences in sessions as fully as possible. Of the 15 patients who came to sessions during this time, five accessed more than three sessions and were willing and able to be interviewed. The boy with whom I had been working following the death of his father, also agreed to be interviewed. In addition to these six interviewees, one patient who had worked with a student music therapist on placement at the hospice also agreed to be interviewed. Several themes, as follows, emerged from the interview transcripts.

Preconceptions and initial impressions

Although one patient had heard other patients talking about their enjoyment of their own sessions, others explained that they had no prior knowledge of what sessions might be like. Several explained that the reality of sessions was different from what they had expected. One had expected music-listening 'like...hypnosis...mystical stuff'; another expected something more like an instrumental lesson, but both were happy with what sessions had been for them. One interviewee had wondered what the therapeutic aspect of the sessions might be, assuming it was not likely to involve 'talking one-to-one' or be something 'you could rub...on', both of which she thought would 'be like therapy'. However, she thought that not knowing in advance had been a good way to go to her first session.

Several patients spoke about their feelings going into their first session. Two spoke of a fear of feeling foolish, and one of these about his initial questioning of the value of the sessions for him, but of his subsequent sense of having benefited in some way:

> I was a bit sceptical...on tenterhooks when I went to my first session...what am I doing here...am I making a mickey out of myself...banging away on a drum... [But] at the end of every session...I've got something out of it...even when I was just playing with the drum and beating.

This patient also spoke of needing time at the start of each of his early sessions to relax and feel less nervous. Another patient, however, described feelings of uncertainty in her first session, but said that she felt more at ease by the third.

A positive effect on mood, a release and a spiritual experience

One patient described how listening to the music as we improvised made him 'feel better in [him]self' and not 'get so hung up'. Another described feeling 'so relieved' after sessions, explaining that it 'takes all of the stress that you have'.

One person valued the opportunity that he found in sessions to 'let himself go', and commented that this was something 'you don't get a chance to do normally'. Another described 'releasing [his] inhibitions' as he played, and described sessions as a place to release internal forces that 'you want to experience...and try and either retrieve or still carry on enjoying'.

Another patient talked about his spirits being lifted and described how he came out of each session on 'a bit of a high'. One interviewee talked of the sense of 'love' and of 'healing' that the sessions brought her; another described the 'peaceful feelings' that he got from improvising with the therapist.

Music therapy sessions and illness

Two patients spoke about the way in which they had felt 'taken out of themselves', causing them to forget their illness and recent hard times, and of this being 'a tremendous boon' to them in their physical or emotional state. One of these two patients referred specifically to being caught up in the experience of active music making with the therapist:

> I think when you play music it's quite different from listening to music. When you play music, you lose yourself into the music. Now I have forgotten to do a tune, but when somebody accompanies me I think you lose yourself into music. There are times when I think I forgot that I was ill, that I had a bad year and things like that.

In talking about the impact of their illness on sessions, one patient described making sessions sometimes shorter than they could otherwise be, due to her feeling unwell. Another patient described his physical exhaustion by the end of sessions. However, he stressed that he kept coming for the experience of 'being taken out of himself', and ascribed his exhaustion in part to his not being well, but also to his having 'worked so hard'.

One patient, who spent his sessions improvising with the therapist, described how the intellectual stimulation that this brought him was helpful for people after a stay in hospital:

> I think...once they come out [of hospital], they're just left at home...you have to find your own way back... It's a way to come back to reality, because you're not in reality when you're in hospital...what you usually do stops...you do nothing...and your brain [is] left...so music is a way...of feeding the brain.

Another patient found intellectual stimulation in learning about the origins and mechanical workings of various unfamiliar instruments.

Sense of potential, purpose and achievement

Two patients spoke of the loss of their singing voice since their illness. One worked on vocal exercises with the therapist to try to improve his range and found pleasure in recovering his voice, 'hearing something normal, that I can do'. The second patient described how he felt held back in sessions because of the hoarseness of his voice. He talked about his sadness that he would never retrieve his singing voice, but explained how, in learning the melody of a favourite song on the piano, he was able to 'sing it in [his] head' as he played.

These two patients also spoke of the focused nature of the work, and of their hopes for the improvements that they would make. One spoke of the sense of purpose that it gave him:

> You've got to concentrate…it does occasionally come. It's frustrating when it doesn't come…but it does give you a purpose… Even though my range is collapsed to a certain extent…I've got a small range that I can work on…and if I work on it…it may be able to improve.

This man also commented that, in attempting to improve the range of his voice in this way, he was overcoming his usual 'defeatist' attitude. The second patient looked forward to the day that he would be able to play the tune he was learning on the piano all the way through, and had made this a clear goal for himself. Other interviewees described feelings of pride and achievement or a sense of having done 'something fruitful'.

Access to musical experience

Some patients described how their musical life had been reduced since their illness. One patient commented that sessions were for her a 'concentrated' form of musical experience. She explained that she now relied on her music therapy sessions for her musical life, as she had stopped listening to music at home since she had become ill. Some patients explained how in music therapy sessions they found access to instruments once again that they had played earlier in their life. Others referred to their enjoyment of the instruments despite not being musically or instrumentally skilled. One explained how playing the instruments had come intuitively to her:

> I don't know how to use the drums, it's just that I think it comes naturally as time goes on… You might be afraid of handling the instruments, or probably not knowing how to use them. I think it's just with trying them out, you tend to love them, then you enjoy them more.

The boy who used his sessions to write a song about his father explained that the sessions brought him something different from other musical 'after-school' activities, saying that they 'added something to his game'. Another man spoke about the difference between listening to music at home and taking part in making music in sessions. He spoke of active music making as a more 'personal thing' than listening, and described 'putting what you feel into that music' as you perform it yourself.

The nature of the relationship, and a sense of partnership

Several interviewees described the non-directive nature of the sessions. One described this as being 'free to do what you want to do, [with the therapist] there as a help and a guide'. This man had been expecting the therapist to take more the role of an instructor, but said that he was happy with sessions being less directive. A patient who had been working on vocal exercises with the therapist commented on his sense that the therapist 'doesn't push you into it', although he admitted sometimes wishing she would.

One interviewee described the sense of partnership he felt as he and I worked together on a song-writing project. Another talked about his enjoyment of the relationship between his playing and that of the therapist, and the way that in his improvising, he could 'link up' with the therapist's playing.

The role and attitude of the music therapist

Several interviewees referred to the music therapist as a 'guide'. One woman valued the moral support she felt in the therapist's accompanying her improvised playing; two patients commented on their valuing the 'feedback' that they got from the therapist as they worked on vocal exercises or learning a melody on the piano. These patients commented on the way that they felt encouraged and 'willed on' by the music therapist. One described the supportive atmosphere that the therapist created:

> She creates an atmosphere that's, I wouldn't say serene, but...I...just feel a sense of...anticipation, presence, which is nice, and...in due course you come out of that shell that I'm in.

Another patient described how the therapist had guided and 'put [him] right' as he 'picked out' a well-known melody on an unfamiliar instrument. This patient also spoke about the way that the therapist's playing enhanced his own improvised playing, describing his admiration of the way that the therapist made 'a little tune out of [his playing]' as he was 'fiddling about...plonking away'.

Music therapy sessions

Exploring family, friends and fellow patients' experiences

A small number of sessions involved a patient's family, friends or fellow patients. To find out more about these people's experiences in sessions, I asked those involved to complete a questionnaire. One respondent was the daughter of a patient with motor neurone disease, who had taken part in her mother's session. She wrote of her happiness in seeing her mother enjoying herself as she played with the therapist, and expressed her gratitude to the therapist for her hard work. She also described her realisation that she could use music to engage with her mother at home.

On one occasion, as I sang quietly to a patient, I became aware of another patient in the bay stopping her conversation with her visitors to listen intently. After I had finished singing, I went over to the lady who had been listening and spoke with her about the session. She talked about how, when she had heard me humming the melody of 'Danny Boy', she had stopped to listen as the melody seemed to come drifting to her from far away. Together with her husband, we then sang the song together. In the questionnaire, she wrote that she had enjoyed being part of the session, and that the song had made her feel 'sentimental'.

On another occasion, the husband of a patient on the ward asked if there was anyone in the hospice who could play some live music for his wife. I took a sounding bowl up to the ward and improvised using that and my voice. I then invited the patient's husband to play with me. The lady lay quietly as we played, smiling when she opened her eyes. When her husband and a friend filled in the questionnaire later on, they described how they had enjoyed having live music in the room and how they had found the session 'peaceful' and 'soothing'. The patient's friend commented that the patient had been 'greatly amused' to see her husband playing the instrument with me, and that the music had created a calm atmosphere in the room and had brought other visitors and patients in the bay together. She also suggested it might be nice to have some live music played outside on a summer's day. The patient's husband, himself a musician, commented on the musical skill and the appropriateness of my playing, and described his pleasure in making progress in his accompanying me in a favourite song. The patient died early the following morning and her husband asked me to play the same instrument at the funeral service, which I did with pleasure.

Exploring staff's experiences and observations

When I worked with patients on the ward, I left feedback forms to be filled in by staff who cared for the patient shortly afterwards. One of the doctors visited a patient who had just spent his first session singing songs he used to sing as a younger man. My colleague commented that the patient's mood appeared 'markedly improved', and wrote that the patient had referred specifically to his music therapy session when talking about his improved mood, saying that he felt 'more himself'. Another patient came to see the music room and, though he was feeling very tired, explored a few of the instruments. A nurse wrote afterwards that the patient had been 'delighted with the idea of music therapy', but that he 'wished he was fitter to enjoy the therapy fully' and that he 'would love to take part again'.

Other nurses were present when I improvised with the husband of a patient on the ward. One of them wrote, as had the patient's husband and friend, of the calming effect of the music. She described how lovely she had found it that other patients in the bay had listened to our playing, and her sense that the session had brought the patients in the bay together in a 'collective activity…which did not require very much of the patients' energy'. Another described the feedback she had from visitors and fellow patients in the bay, who had not been disturbed, but had enjoyed the music and the sounds of laughter and enjoyment in the room. This staff member also attended the funeral of this patient, and observed many people approaching me afterwards to say how much they appreciated my playing as a tribute to the patient, and how they had found the music moving and interesting.

On two occasions, I had feedback from staff after they had observed or taken part in slightly different musical events. The first was the birthday celebration of the son of a patient on the ward. The nurses knew that the patient's family were musical and asked if I could go and make some music with them in the patient's room. I could not go on the birthday itself, but left some instruments with the nurses. The patient and family invited staff in to celebrate with them, and they all played the instruments as they sang 'Happy Birthday'. The nurses later described how they had all 'made a lot of noise, which brought laughter into the room and everyone enjoyed the occasion'. They added that though the patient was now dying, they hoped the family would have happy memories of her son's birthday. On the second occasion, the daughter of a patient came to the day unit and asked if she could play the piano that was there. My colleague listened as she played and later wrote that she felt the girl had valued the opportunity to come away from the intensity of the room where her mother was dying and express how she was feeling. She felt that the girl had appreciated the space given to her to do this in her own way. My colleague also wondered whether it would be a good idea to have some instruments positioned around the hospice, where patients, staff and visitors who wished to make some 'spontaneous sound – musical or otherwise!' could do so.

Exploring perceptions of music therapy amongst the broader staff team

In order to explore perceptions of music therapy amongst clinical staff across the hospice, I selected at random a number of staff from each clinical department to answer a questionnaire, for example, nursing staff on each of the four wards, nursing staff in the day unit, the social work and welfare team. I gave out 25 questionnaires; 17 were returned completed, and a further two were returned partially completed. The questions and a summary of the responses are described below.

What is your understanding of what happens in music therapy sessions, and the part these sessions can play as an aspect of specialist palliative care?

Most responses to this question concerned the benefit that staff felt music therapy sessions held for patients. The most frequent responses referred to an opportunity for the expression or release of emotion, and for non-verbal communication. Staff also spoke of spiritual or uplifting effects of music and the positive influence of music therapy sessions on patients' mood. Some commented on the possibilities for a patient to explore his own creativity, and others on the value of sessions in combating a sense of monotony. Two spoke of the potential for sessions to reduce a patient's sense of isolation, one commented on the potential for patients to gain a sense of achievement, and another on the value of music as a distraction from pain. Whilst most comments seemed to be based on an understanding of music therapy sessions as active participation in music making, one person commented that listening to music offers patients a non-physical involvement in therapeutic activity.

Several staff described their impressions of what took place in sessions. Most referred to spontaneous music making or singing, some to music listening, and one to the use of music in legacy projects. Some staff stated their understanding that sessions usually took place on a one-to-one basis, while a few mentioned that sessions might include family, friends and staff, or larger groups. Some referred to the collaborative nature of music making in sessions and the way that sessions are patient-led. Six referred to a supportive and empathic relationship being established between the patient and music therapist.

What has influenced your views?

For most staff, it was their own experiences of music that influenced their views. Several others described having had feedback from patients and their families or from colleagues who had cared for patients referred to sessions. Some staff mentioned formal presentations of music therapy they had been to, informal discussions with me, or overhearing me introducing the idea of music therapy to patients. A few staff had worked with music therapists in other organisations, or had witnessed a music therapy session.

Have you ever referred patients to music therapy sessions?

While seven staff had referred patients to music therapy sessions, 12 had not. Staff were also asked if they had referred patients to other aspects of the Creative Living Centre: 16 of the 17 staff had, although two of these seemed to be referrals to general activity in the day unit. Reasons for referral to music therapy included a patient's love of or interest in music, with one person refering a patient with a now limited access to this interest; a patient's physiological or emotional limitations in expression or communication; a desire for the patient to be actively creative; and a perceived need for a non-threatening medium in which a patient could explore feelings of conflict and frustration.

The most frequent reason given for not referring patients was a lack of understanding of music therapy. Slightly less frequently, staff wrote that they had not thought that patients they worked with would have benefited from sessions, or were not aware, or only recently aware, of music therapy being available. Two said that they tended to 'signpost' patients, giving them details of what was available at the hospice, then letting the patient identify something they would be interested in. A complementary therapist commented that referrals to psychological therapies were usually made by the home care teams before the patient reached her service. As in the case of referrals to the Creative Living Centre as a whole, one staff member explained that she just did not think about referring to music therapy.

Is there anything you feel would helpfully inform your understanding of music therapy in specialist palliative care?

Staff commented here on information content and forms of information presentation. Most said they would like to attend a teaching seminar, or attend or assist in a session. One person preferred information leaflets. On information content, most staff sought either 'general information', to learn the value and benefits of music therapy, or to understand what sessions involve at a practical level. One staff member wrote that she would like to learn more about appropriate referral criteria, one that she would like to hear case studies of work with patients, and one that she would like to know more about the difference between 'music' and 'music therapy'. Another requested regular reminders of services available to patients.

Music-making groups

Experiences of patients and observations of staff

As an occasional alternative to the usual weekly group activities, I held a music-making group in the day unit or the garden pavilion. Sometimes, we used percussion instruments and our voices to improvise music together, sometimes recording the group and listening back afterwards to the music we had made. One or two patients asked for copies of these recordings, which they were able to have on CD. On one occasion, I encouraged the patients to use the instruments to conjure up sounds of something that was important to them, such as a favourite pastime, a holiday or a memory from childhood, which we then talked about. At other times we sang songs.

After a session of improvised music making, I gathered comments from the staff who had been present or who had seen patients later that day. These staff commented often on patients' enjoyment and interaction in the group, and particularly on the participation of some patients who were usually more withdrawn:

> T…had fun, he was involved. He's usually very quiet and reserved, but…when it was time to go home, he got up and said, 'I'm going home now. 'Bye everyone!' He was a changed man!

Another activity was 'musical bingo'. In this, we combined bingo-type score-cards with song sheets; each number corresponded to a song on the sheet. When a number was picked out, and whoever had that number on their score-card had ticked it off, patients and staff joined together in singing that song. After two such groups on different days, a colleague asked the groups to answer a few questions about their experiences.

All spoke of enjoying the sessions, using words such as 'pleasant' and 'up-lifting'. One said that participating in the music helped to 'forget about what you are suffering'; another found it 'a way of releasing if you're feeling a bit stressed or you're angry about something'. Several spoke about the sense of 'ca-maraderie' or 'togetherness' that they felt in the group, and others described how it had reminded them of singing these songs at family parties or in child-hood days. Others had been motivated to listen to music when they got home later that afternoon. Patients appreciated the flexibility of the musical aspect of the game, for example, the option to 'sit…and listen and clap and tap your feet to the music if they did not want to join in'. Some liked the excitement and anticipation added to the singing activity by the 'bingo'.

Patients also had ideas for future sessions. Some wanted an 'open mic' session, taking turns to perform; others suggested having a pre-session drink, 'like we're actually outside in a theatre'. One man suggested the group worked on a project, then invited family and friends for a 'mini-concert'. Another, however, preferred not to invite others in, as being 'on show' might make him 'more…conservative in outlook'.

Concerts and live entertainment

I coordinated many live music events in the hospice during the evaluation period, including performances by professional and amateur musicians, children and adults. Once, a staff member performed a programme of folk music. Concerts were advertised to patients, staff and visitors, and I asked audiences to answer a questionnaire. A colleague interviewed the staff member who performed.

Many respondents described enjoying the concert, saying it made a change to their daily routine. Some talked of its being 'relaxing' or 'comforting'. One wrote that the concert had 'cheered him up', while another found that a particular song brought back memories of difficult times and made her 'a touch sad'. One person described his enjoyment of the more lively pieces but would have preferred some shorter pieces between the longer ones. Several patients looked forward to future concerts, and one commented that she would 'go home wanting to listen to music more often'.

A common theme among non-clinical staff's comments was pleasure in this rare opportunity to 'mingle with patients and relatives'. Some enjoyed hearing music drifting down the hallway when they could not attend the concert, making 'paperwork more pleasant', while others commented on the event being 'a nice way to start an afternoon's work'. One person was delighted seeing a patient she had thought could not walk, get up and dance, and decided to spend more time listening to music. Another person appreciated the concert being held in the chapel, saying: 'it gave the event a special feel'. She also suggested a daily opportunity for staff to listen to music for relaxation and meditation.

One staff member was interested to see 'another side' to the staff member who performed. The staff member who performed spoke of his gratitude for his job as a steward at the hospice, and his pleasure in being able to 'give something back'. He thought it healthy to contribute to the social environment of the hospice outside normal day-to-day responsibilities. He appreciated the way in which music can evoke memories in listeners, and believed that people connect easily with folk music because of the every-day nature of its lyrics. Most strongly, he conveyed his sense of privilege and delight in sharing music he loved with an attentive audience that included many patients.

Summary

This study explored the experiences of patients, patients' friends and families and staff of the many aspects of the music and music therapy service at St Christopher's Hospice. Patients accessing music therapy sessions described a number of positive outcomes, including improved mood, a distraction from illness and a sense of purpose and achievement; families had observed patients' enjoyment of sessions and had themselves benefited from being involved. Those accessing group sessions expressed the sense of camaraderie they felt; staff commented on the active involvement of patients usually more isolated from others. Feedback gathered at concerts indicated the enjoyment of patients and staff alike. A non-clinical staff member who performed indicated his sense of privilege at being able to bring something of value to patients and contribute to the social life of the hospice in this way.

The study also explored clinical staff's perceptions of the use of music therapy in adult palliative care, and gathered their views on effective ways of promoting awareness of the service amongst staff.

The results form a valuable contribution to a growing evidence base for the role and value of music therapy within palliative care. They present the experiences and opinions of those accessing and referring to the service, and support existing literature written from the viewpoint of music therapists.

Further reading

Aldridge, D. (ed.) (1998) *Music Therapy in Palliative Care: New Voices.* London: Jessica Kingsley Publishers.

A selection of music therapists describe their work in various palliative care settings, working with children and adults with different approaches and in different countries.

Lee, C. (ed.) (1994) *Lonely Waters: Proceedings of the International Conference Music Therapy in Palliative Care.* Oxford: Sobell.

This book includes the proceedings from the international conference Music Therapy in Palliative Care, Oxford, in 1994. The contributors are all specialists and address issues that are relevant to music therapists, healthcare professionals and those interested in the use of music with the dying.

Munro, S. (1984) *Music Therapy in Palliative/Hospice Care.* Boulevard, St Louis, MO: Magnamusic-Baton, Inc.

An overview of providing music therapy in palliative care settings in the USA.

15 Conclusion

Malcolm Payne and Nigel Hartley

This book makes a case for the role of creative arts in palliative care. In this concluding chapter, we set out a summary of our argument. Much of the force of the argument for creative arts in palliative care is contained in the chapters of Part II where artists and craftspeople express how they do their work and what it means to them and their patients.

We started out by claiming in Chapter 1 a number of potential roles for the creative arts:

- Since creative work is a vital human activity, a palliative care that seeks to help people live until the moment that they die must include the arts as part of its work. Any human activity, if it is vital, must be represented in people's life experience right up to the end of life.

- Art and creative work enhances psychological and social stability, enriches human life and enables people to experience self-fulfilment in creation.

- Art and creative work enables patients and families to find solace and relief from distress and difficulty.

- The arts can be an instrument of psychological therapy.

The creative arts may be offered to patients and their carers in a wide range of settings:

- day care, the traditional centre for arts and creative work
- inpatient units and hospitals, at the bedside and in other spaces that permit group and family work

- community settings or drop-in centres where people meet to respond to the difficulties of their illness
- GP surgeries, healthy living centres and other healthcare settings
- care homes.

The arts facilitate communication where it is physically, socially or psychologically difficult. Participation and inclusion through creative work can enable patients and their families to repair relationships among themselves when facing the stress of an advanced and final illness. Freeing people up to express the inexpressible or difficult to express, or to express the value of diverse lifestyles and life experiences, can also develop from creative experiences. Where people have learning disabilities or dementia, creative experiences, even of a simple kind such as participation in shared music making, can permit inclusion in human interaction. Patients whose lives seem out of control because they are being taken over by an illness that is hard to manage can at least gain control over creative materials to produce an artistic product that incorporates something of themselves, memories, and values that they hold important.

The consequence of these possibilities is that a comprehensive arts service in palliative care might include:

- arts therapies
- arts facilitation
- community arts.

However, making all these possibilities available through professional artists is not always viable for a smaller hospice or a palliative care service restricted by its role in, say, a hospital or care home setting. Volunteer work and sessional or occasional provision can still make a valid contribution to the holistic experience of a palliative care service.

Among important practice principles in palliative care arts work are:

- offering choice in activity and materials
- helping people share experiences and support each other through working together creatively, both helping each other and joining shared projects
- exhibiting and giving art objects created through arts work to friends and family is an important motivator
- focusing on patients' responses, feelings and motivation in working creatively
- taking care, through interaction with patients and carers, and through research, audit and evaluation as part of practice, to gain feedback to inform the service of what works, what helps and what hinders.

All these processes must be carefully managed. A clear understanding of the objectives that any particular arts service aims to meet is a crucial part of providing an effective arts service in palliative care. Connected to that understanding, management decisions can be made about the selection of service focuses among the possibilities discussed in this book. Managing the service will require the setting up of appropriate management and supervision arrangements and using human resources, artists, volunteers and other staff, appropriately to achieve those outcomes. Another important management task is articulating a vision of the contribution of the arts in any particular palliative care service and connecting it forcefully with the objectives of the overall service.

In the model of arts provision outlined in Chapter 1 (Figure 1.1), we drew attention to the interaction of patient, family and community with the artists in their organisation and with each other. Thinking about the intended interrelationships among these parties and helping people build interactions through their involvement in arts and creative work will help the service achieve its objectives in contributing to the holistic palliative care service. To go beyond this, patients' and artists' achievements can be a powerful representative of palliative care and its work in the community and a message of the value of the arts in society generally and in healthcare.

There are many opportunities in palliative care practice to help people in great pain and distress at the end of their lives and to develop the arts. We are committed to extending those opportunities and we hope we have shared that commitment in this book in a way that will encourage you to join with us.

Bibliography

Addington-Hall, J., Bruera, E., Higginson, I.J. and Payne, S. (eds) (2007) *Research Methods in Palliative Care*. Oxford: Oxford University Press.

Aldridge, D. (ed.) (1998) *Music Therapy in Palliative Care: New Voices*. London: Jessica Kingsley Publishers.

Ansdell, G. (1995) *Music For Life*. London: Jessica Kingsley Publishers.

Ansdell, G. and Hartley, N. (2000) 'The legacy of music therapy'(Abstract) *The programme of the Annual Conference of the Association of Professional Music therapists and the British Society for Music Therapy*, February.

Ansdell, G. and Pavlicevic, M. (2001) *Beginning Research in the Arts Therapies: A Practical Guide*. London: Jessica Kingsley Publishers.

Armstrong, M. (2006) *A Handbook of Human Resource Management Practice* (10th edn). London: Kogan Page.

Artlink (2005) *Extraordinary Everyday: Further Explorations in Collaborative Art in Health Care*. Edinburgh: Artlink.

Atrill, P. and McLaney, E. (2004) *Accounting and Finance for Non-Specialists* (4th edn). Upper Saddle River, NJ: Prentice Hall.

Bell, S. (1998) 'Art Therapy in the Community.' In M. Pratt and M. Wood (eds) *Art Therapy in Palliative Care*. London: Routledge.

Bernhard, R. (1979) *Collecting Light: The Photographs of Ruth Bernhard*. Carmel, CA: The Friends of Photography.

Blake, W. (1977) *The Complete Poems*, ed. A. Ostriker. Harmondsworth: Penguin.

Bolton, G. and Hedges, D. (2005) *Poetry, Therapy and Emotional Life*. Oxford: Radcliffe.

Bunting, C. (2007) *Public Value and the Arts in England*. London: Arts Council England.

Case, C. and Dalley, T. (1992) *The Handbook of Art Therapy*. London: Routledge.

Casement, P. (2002) *Learning from our Mistakes. Beyond Dogma in Psychoanalysis and Psychotherapy*. London: Brunner Routledge.

Connell, C. (1992) 'Art therapy as part of the palliative care programme.' *Palliative Medicine 6*, 18–25.

Connell, C. (1994) *Something Understood: Art Therapy in Cancer Care*. London: Wrexham.

deMong S.A. (1997) 'Provision of recreational activities in hospices in the United States.' *The Hospice Journal 12*, 4, 57–67.

Douglas, H., Normand, C., Higginson, I. and Goodwin, D. (2003) 'Palliative day care: What does it cost to run a centre and does attendance affect use of other services?' *Palliative Medicine 17*, 628–37.

Emery, A.E. (1997) 'Medicine, artists and their art.' *Journal of the Royal College of Physicians of London 31*, 4, 350–5.

Foucault, M. (1986) *The Foucault Reader*. Harmondsworth: Penguin.

Gibson, A. (1995) 'Creativity in hospice – a celebration of achievement.' *Occupational Therapy News*, June, 4–5.

Gill, S. and Fox, J. (2004) *The Dead Good Funerals Book*. Carlisle: Engineers of the Imagination.

Hart, C. (1998) *Doing a Literature Review: Releasing the Social Science Research Imagination*. London: Sage.

Hart, C. (2001) *Doing a Literature Search: A Comprehensive Guide for the Social Sciences*. London: Sage.

Hartley, N.A. (2001) 'On a personal note: A music therapist's reflections on working with those who are living with a terminal illness.' *Journal of Palliative Care 17*, 3, 135–41.

Hartley, N. (2005) 'Love…Actually? – Attempting to Aticulate the Heart of Hospice.' In C. Dileo and J. Loewy (eds) *Music Therapy at the End of Life*. Cherry Hill, NJ: Jeffrey Books.

Hartley N. (2007) 'Resilience and Creativity.' In B. Monroe and D. Oliviere (eds) *Resilience in Palliative Care* Oxford: Oxford University Press.

Higginson, I.J., Hearn, J., Myers, K. and Naysmith, A. (2000) 'Palliative day care: What do services do?' *Palliative Medicine 14*, 4, 277–86.

Hogan, B.E. (2003) 'Soul music in the twilight years: Music therapy and the dying process.' *Topics in Geriatric Rehabilitation 19*, 4, 275–79.

Johnson, G., Scholes, K. and Whittington, R. (2005) *Exploring Corporate Strategy* (7th edn). Upper Saddle River, NJ: Prentice Hall.

Kaye, P. (1998) 'Some Images of Illness.' In M. Pratt and M. Wood (eds) *Art Therapy in Palliative Care*. London: Routledge.

Kearney, M. (2000) *A Place of Healing*. Oxford: Oxford University Press.

Kennett, C. (2000) 'Participation in a creative arts project can foster hope in a hospice day centre.' *Palliative Medicine 14*, 5, 419–25.

Kennett C. (2001) 'Psychosocial Day Care.' In J. Hearn and M. Myers (eds) *Palliative Day Care in Practice*. Oxford: Oxford University Press.

Kennett, C., Harmer, L. and Tasker, M. (2004) 'Bringing the arts to the bedside.' *European Journal of Palliative Care 11*, 6, 254–6.

Knight, K. and Schwarzman, M. (2005) *Beginners Guide to Community-Based Arts*. Oakland, CA: New Village Press.

Kübler-Ross, E. (1970) *On Death and Dying*. London: Tavistock.

Learmonth, M. and Huckvale, K. (2002) 'A gap in the Arts.' Available from: www.Insiderart.org.uk/ userfiles/file/A%20Gap%20in%20the%20arts.pdf (accessed on 29 October 2007).

Lee, C. (ed.) (1994) *Lonely Waters: Proceedings of the International Conference Music Therapy in Palliative Care*. Oxford: Sobell.

Lee, C. (1996) *Music at the Edge: the Music Therapy Experiences of a Musician Living with AIDS*. London: Routledge.

McLouglin, D. (1995) 'Creative writing in hospice.' *Hospice Bulletin*, October: 8–9.

McLoughlin, D. (1997) 'Teaching writing in a hospice day centre.' *Writing in Education 11* (Spring), 7–9.

McNiff, S. (1992) *Art as Medicine, Creating a Therapy of the Imagination*. London: Piatkus.

Magee, W. (2000) 'Dialogues: A response to the review of *Music Therapy in Palliative Care – New Voices*.' *British Journal of Music Therapy 14*, 2, 93–4.

Marcel, G. (1995) *The Philosophy of Existentialism*. Washington, DC: Citadel Press.

Marrone, M. (1998) *Attachment and Interaction*. London: Jessica Kingsley Publishers.

Mintzberg, H., Ahlstrand, B. and Lampel, J. (1998) *Strategy Safari – the Complete Guide Through the Wilds of Strategic Management*. Upper Saddle River, NJ: Prentice Hall.

Munro, S. (1984) *Music Therapy in Palliative/Hospice Care.* Boulevard, St Louis, MO: Magnamusic-Baton, Inc.

O'Callaghan, C. (1996) 'Complementary therapies in terminal care: Pain, music creativity and music therapy in palliative care.' *The American Journal of Hospice and Palliative Care,* March/April, 43–9.

Payne, M. (2006) 'Social objectives in cancer care: the example of palliative day care.' *European Journal of Cancer Care 15,* 440–7.

Petrone, M.A. (1997) *The Emotional Cancer Journey.* Brighton: ESBH Health Authority.

Pratt, A. and Thomas, G. (2002) *Guidelines for Arts Therapists and the Arts in Palliative Care Settings.* London: Hospice Information.

Pratt, M. and Wood, M.J.M. (1998) *Art Therapy in Palliative Care: the Creative Response.* London: Routledge.

Robson, C. (2002) *Real World Research* (2nd edn). Oxford: Blackwell.

Rogers, C. (2003) *Client Centred Therapy* (new edn). London: Constable.

Ronaldson, S. (1997) '*Terminally old.*' Paper presented at the National Hospice and Palliative Care Association Conference, Canberra.

Rosetta Life (2007) www.rosettalife.org (accessed on 30 January 2008).

Salmon, D. (2001) 'Music therapy as psychospiritual process in palliative care.' *Journal of Palliative Care 17,* 3, 142–7.

Schaverien, J. (1998) *The Revealing Image.* London: Jessica Kingsley Publishers.

Senior, P. and Croall, J. (1993) *Helping to Heal: Arts in Health Care.* London: Calouste Gulbenkian Foundation.

Shaw, B. (1999) '"Parting gifts": Palliative care patients' perceptions of making sculptures.' *Palliative Care Today 8,* 3, 36–7.

Sheikh, A.A. (2003) *Healing Images: The Role of Imagination in Health.* Amityville NY: Baywood.

Spencer, D.J. and Daniels, L.E. (1998) 'Day hospice care – a review of the literature.' *Palliative Medicine 12,* 4, 219–29.

Stanworth, R. (2003) *Recognising Spiritual Needs in People who are Dying.* Oxford: Oxford University Press.

Thomas, G. (1995) 'Art therapy and practice in palliative care.' *European Journal of Palliative Care 2,* 3, 120–1.

Volunteering England (2007) *Guidelines for relations between volunteers and paid workers in the Health and Personal Social Services.* Available at www.volunteering.org.uk/Resources/publications/ Guidelines+for+relations+between+volunteers+and+paid+workers+in+the+Health+and+ Personal+Social+Servi.htm (accessed on 26 October 2007)

Walker-Kuhne, D. (2005) *Invitation to the Party: Building Bridges to the Arts, Culture and Community.* New York: Theatre Communications Group.

Waller, D. (2002) *Art Therapies and Progressive Illness: Nameless Dread.* Hove: Brunner-Routledge.

Waller, D. and Sibbett, C. (eds) (2005) *Facing Death: Art Therapy and Cancer Care.* Buckingham: Open University Press.

Whittington, R. (2000) *What is Strategy and Does it Matter?* (2nd edn). London: Thomson.

Windsor, J. (2007) *Your Health and the Arts.* London: Arts Council England.

Winnicott, D. (1971) *Playing and Reality.* London: Tavistock/Routledge.

Yalom, I. (1998) *The Gift of Therapy: Reflections on Being a Therapist.* London: Piatkus.

Contributors

Adrian Butchers

Adrian started working at St Christopher's 17 years ago to help set up and run the new salon that was being opened to provide a hairdressing service for patients on the inpatient unit and those attending the day centre. In the past he owned two salons of his own and with a partner also ran a catering business specialising in wedding receptions. During that time he trained in the art of sugar craft and went on to design and make wedding and celebration cakes. Having always had an interest in arts and crafts he attended several different college courses to learn a new range of different skills, including mosaics and silk painting, and 7 years ago joined the arts team at the hospice to teach a wide range of crafts to the patients on the wards, day centre and in the community.

Tamsin Dives

Tamsin Dives trained initially at the Guildhall School of Music, gaining the AGSM in 1982. For 22 years she pursued a diverse career as an opera and concert singer. In 2005 she returned to the Guildhall to retrain as a music therapist. Since qualifying she has worked with adults with severe learning difficulties, challenging behaviour and brain injury. She has served on the BSMT committee. She now works as a music therapist at St Christopher's Hospice and also with primary school children with emotional and behavioural problems.

Samantha Dobbs

Samantha Dobbs is art psychotherapist at St Christopher's Hospice, and artist and nurse health adviser at Chichester University. Samantha trained at Goldsmiths University London 2004 – 2006 and has worked at the hospice since qualifying. She is interested in attachment theory and Jungian psychonalysis. She plans to work with children in the hospice environment and also in learning difficulties and mainstream schools. Sam originally trained as a Registered General Nurse in 1992.

Abi Gill

Abi trained as a music therapist at the Nordoff-Robbins Music Therapy Centre in London, qualifying in 2004. She introduced the music therapy service at St Christopher's Hospice, working there for two and a half years before moving on to develop a music therapy service working with adults with epilepsy at the National Society for Epilepsy in Buckinghamshire.

Lynn Harmer

Lynn Harmer is one of the arts team at St Christopher's Hospice and a lecturer in art and ceramics at Greenwich Community College in South London. Having trained as a teacher and counsellor she has worked in a wide variety of healthcare settings as well as having her own ceramic studio in both Devon and South London. She is one of the contributors to the article 'Bringing the Arts to the Bedside' (*European Journal of Palliative Care* (2004) *11*, 6, 254–26).

Nigel Hartley

Nigel Hartley currently holds the post of Director of Supportive Care at St Christopher's Hospice, London. He has worked in end-of-life care for the past eighteen years, more recently working on the redevelopment of Day Services at St Christopher's Hospice before taking on his current position. He has held posts at both London Lighthouse, a centre for those living with HIV/AIDS, and also Sir Michael Sobell House, which is a large hospice in Oxford. He is an experienced manager, counsellor, musician, community musician, and music therapist.

He has chaired both the Association of Professional Music Therapists (UK) and the British Society of Music Therapy, and has sat on the Allied Health Professions Forum as an Arts Therapies representative. In 2002, he chaired the organising committee for the 10th World Congress of Music Therapy which was held in the UK.

Nigel's main interests and passions are based around how we listen in our lives, and the language that we use to articulate our relationship experiences. Nigel has a national and international reputation as a teacher in end-of-life care and he regularly publishes about his work.

Virginia Hearth

Gini Hearth is a community artist at St Christopher's Hospice, visual artist and integrative arts psychotherapist in training. She has worked in a variety of community contexts and organisations including prisons, refuges, hostels for homeless people, probation services, psychiatric wards, drug and alcohol addictions clinics, nursing homes, schools and colleges. She has worked on projects with asylum seekers and refugees, looked-after children, carers, deaf and disabled people and families. She uses a wide range of arts practices to devise collaborative projects either for groups or individual work.

Malcolm Payne

Malcolm Payne is Director, Psychosocial and Spiritual Care, St Christopher's Hospice, and Honorary Professor, Kingston University/St George's University of London. He has worked in probation, social services and the national and local voluntary sector and university posts, being for many years Professor and Head of Applied Community Studies, Manchester Metropolitan University. He is the author of many books and articles, including *Modern Social Work Theory* (3rd edn, Palgrave Macmillan 2006), *What is Professional Social Work?* (2nd edn, Policy Press 2006) and *Teamwork in Multiprofessional Care* (Palgrave Macmillan 2000), and as editor (with Steven Shardlow) of *Social Work in the British Isles* (Jessica Kingsley Publishers 2002).

Mick Sands

Mick Sands has a degree in English and American Literature from the University of Manchester and a P.G.C.S.E. from the University of London. He taught English in secondary schools in London and then worked for an international charity which helps create communities with people with a learning difficulty – L'Arche – and was the director of the Lambeth community of L'Arche for six years. He has been working in classical theatre as a composer since 1989. He is a winner of the Christopher Whelan award for music in theatre and in 2001 was nominated for an EMMY for his score for a television documentary on American PBS. He has worked with adults with a learning difficulty using music and drama since the 1970s. He is a traditional singer/musician whose first solo CD "The Ominous and the Luminous" was released in 2007.

Marion Tasker

Marion Tasker trained at Ravensbourne College of Art and Design studying technical and botanical illustration. She worked in audiovisual design and then as an illustrator in medical publishing. She went freelance in 1990 and her clients include Elsevier, Taylor and Francis, Butterworth Heinemann, Harper Collins, Greycoat Publishing, Spires Design, Binary Vision, Designers Collective. She currently works part-time at St Christopher's Hospice as a community artist.

Suppliers

Art, crafts, design materials

Craft Creations
Telephone: 01992 781900; fax: 01992 634339; email: enquiries@craftcreations.com; website: www.craftcreations.co.uk, accessed on 19 February 2008.

Craft Creations provides a mail order service and has a very large range of blank and aperture cards and a wide range of accessories for card making.

Great Art
Gerstaecker UK Ltd, Normandy House, 1 Nether Street, Alton, Hampshire, GU34 1EA

Telephone: 0845 601 5772/01420 59 3332; fax: 01420 59 3333; email: welcome@greatart.co.uk

IKEA
IKEA local stores may be found in many parts of the country.

UK website: www.ikea.com/gb/en, accessed on 19 February 2008.

Jacksons Arts Supplies
1 Farleigh Place, London N16 7SX

Telephone: 0870 241 1849; fax: 0870 770 0360; website: www.jacksonart.co.uk

Kent County Supplies
PO Box 196, West Malling, Kent ME19 6PX

Telephone: 0845 270 8811; fax: 0800 243 732; email: ksales@kent.gov.uk

Lakeland
Lakeland's Craft Creative website: www.lakeland.co.uk/category.aspx/crafts, accessed on 19 February 2008. Local stores may be found in many parts of the country.

Specialist Crafts Ltd
PO Box 247, Leicester LE1 9QS

Telephone: 0116 269 0959; fax: 0116 269 7722; email: info@specialistcrafts.co.uk; website: www.specialistcrafts.co.uk, accessed on 19 February 2008.

Felt-making

Wingham Wool Work
70 Main St, Wentworth, Rotherham, South Yorkshire S62 7TN

Telephone: 01226 742926; fax: 01226 741166; email: wingwool@clara.net

Framing

Wessex Pictures

2b Beddington Lane Industrial Estate, 117 Beddington Lane, Croydon, Surrey CR0 4TD

Telephone: 020 8683 0055; fax: 0208 6831123; email: sales@wessexpictures.com

Mosaics

Mosaic Workshop

Workshop – Holloway, Unit B, 443–449 Holloway Road, London N7 6LJ

Telephone/fax: 020 7272 2446

Shop – Holborn, 1a Princeton Street, London WC1R 4AX

Telephone: 020 7831 0889; email: sales@mosaicworkshop.com. website: www.mymosaicworkshop.co.uk/index.html, accessed on 19 February 2008.

Music

LMS Music Suppliers

PO Box 7, Exeter EX1 1WB

Telephone: 0845 230 0455; fax: 01392 412521; email: LMSmusic@compuserve.com; website: www.LMSmusicsupplies.co.uk, accessed on 19 February 2008.

Sounding Bowls

Tobias Kaye, The Workshop, 11 Lower Dean, Buckfastleigh, Devon TQ11 0LS

Telephone/fax: 01364 642 837; email: Tobias@TobiasKaye.co.uk; website: www.SoundingBowls.com, accessed on 19 February 2008.

Pottery

PotteryCrafts Ltd

Cambell Road, Stoke on Trent ST4 4ET

Telephone: 01782 746000; fax: 01782 746000; email: sales@potterycrafts.co.uk

Potters Connection Ltd

Chadwick Street, Longton, Stoke on Trent ST3 1PJ

Telephone: 01782 598729; fax: 01782 593054; email: sales@potters-connection.sagehost.co.uk, accessed on 19 February 2008.

Sculpture

Alec Tiranti Ltd

3 Piper Court, Berkshire Drive, Thatcham, Berkshire RG19 4ER

Telephone: 0845 123 2100; fax: 0845 123 2101; website: www.tiranti.co.uk, accessed on 19 February 2008.

South Western Industrial Plasters

63 Netherstreet, Bromham, Chippenham, Wiltshire SN15 2DP

Telephone: 01380 850616; fax: 01380 859638

Silk painting

Rainbow Silks

6 Wheelers Yard, High Street, Great Missenden, Bucks HP16 0AL

Mail order 01494 862111; shop: 01494 862929; fax: 01494 862651; email: caroline@rainbowsilks.co.uk; website: www.rainbowsilks.co.uk/index.cfm, accessed on 19 February 2008.

Strong tissue paper – 'wet strength'

Richards and Appleby

Unit 3, Heads of the Valley Industrial Estate, Rhymney, Gwent NP22 5RL

Telephone: 01685 843384; fax: 01685 842466

Templates, art books

Search Press

Wellwood, North Farm Road, Tunbridge Wells, Kent TN2 3DR

Telephone: 01892 510850; website: www.searchpress.com, accessed on 19 February 2008.

Withies, willow sticks

J Burdekins Ltd

Wakefield Road, Osset WF5 9AQ

Telephone: 01924 273103; fax: 01924 265921; email: sales@jburdekin.co.uk

P.H. Coates & Sons

Mare Green, Stoke St. Gregory, Nr Taunton, Somerset TA3 6HY

Telephone: 01823 490249; fax: 01823 490814; email: phcoate@globalnet.co.uk

Subject Index

Author Index